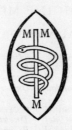

MIND & MEDICINE MONOGRAPHS

Editor

MICHAEL BALINT, M.D., PH.D., M.SC.

18

Motherhood and Personality

Motherhood and Personality

Psychosomatic Aspects of Childbirth

LÉON CHERTOK

with

M. BONNAUD

M. BORELLI   J-L. DONNET

C. REVAULT D'ALLONNES

Foreword by Norman Morris

TAVISTOCK PUBLICATIONS

J. B. LIPPINCOTT COMPANY

First published in Great Britain in 1969
by Tavistock Publications Limited
11 New Fetter Lane, London E C 4
Printed in Great Britain
in 10 pt Times, 2 pt leaded
by Spottiswoode, Ballantyne & Co Ltd
London and Colchester
This translation © Tavistock Publications Limited, 1969

Translation by D. Graham

SBN 422 71880 7

Originally published in French under the title
Féminité et Maternité
by Desclée De Brouwer, Paris
© Desclée De Brouwer, 1966

Distributed in the United States of America and in Canada by
J. B. Lippincott Company, Philadelphia and Toronto

Contents

Figures and Tables

Foreword

Preparation for childbirth is now widely practised throughout the world. In general, European obstetricians and psychiatrists have shown more interest in this important subject than their colleagues in other continents. France in particular has been associated with many notable studies and has several centres that are now well famed for their significant observations. It is therefore not surprising that this remarkable new publication should have been written by a French psychiatrist whose research studies in this field are already very well known.

For too long the psychological problems associated with pregnancy and childbirth have received far too little attention from obstetricians and psychiatrists. Various methods of preparation for childbirth have, however, been developed during recent years. Often these programmes have appeared to rest on dogmatic assumptions and improper claims. Very little attempt has been made to explain the psychological principles on which they are based. Support for these different methods often seems to reflect a 'religious-like' enthusiasm rather than an impartial, objective, scientific appraisal, and, as a result, many obstetricians have tended to suspect the claims that have been made. This situation has therefore constituted a major obstacle to the expansion and development of these important techniques.

Léon Chertok in this present book has attempted to explore in far greater detail than ever before the various psychological theories on which preparation for childbirth is based. This is a field in which he has had considerable experience for many years, and I know of no other author so suited to this extremely difficult task. He has completed a most comprehensive review of the literature, much of which until now has never really received consideration in such depth. To this invaluable analysis he has added reports of his own very important research studies.

In my view this book will prove of enormous interest and value to all those who, like myself, are concerned in this subject. It sets a new standard of appraisal and assessment that will do much to remove the

Motherhood and Personality

remaining scepticism and reaction which have been difficult finally to uproot because of our limited knowledge and scientific data.

I am certain that this study by Léon Chertok will prove to be a standard work of reference for many years to come. In many senses it represents a milestone in the evolution of this subject. I am both honoured and proud to have been asked to write this foreword.

My only reservation is that these words of mine do not match the quality of scholarship which this book deserves.

NORMAN MORRIS, M.D., F.R.C.O.G.
Professor of Obstetrics and Gynaecology
Charing Cross Hospital Medical School
July 1968

Preface

In 1958, thanks to a grant from the Foundations Fund for Research in Psychiatry, I was able to embark upon a project of research on pain in childbirth and psychological analgesia. For several years I had been interested in psychosomatic problems, and it had occurred to me that childbirth, involving biological, psychological, and social factors, was a psychosomatic act *par excellence*. I was interested in the ways in which emotional factors might be related to both the physiology of childbirth and the pain involved. This last appeared to offer a particularly good field for research, since childbirth is a general phenomenon, accessible to observation, non-pathological, and predictable in advance. It provides a more or less uniform anatomical and physiological substratum, while the amount of pain experienced varies. It is also an event of great emotional significance in the woman's life. Finally, I felt that a better understanding of the pain of childbirth should throw light on some aspects of the recalcitrant problem of pain in general. A decade ago I embarked upon a study of the theoretical and practical problems in the methods of prepared childbirth. I then decided that a thorough understanding of psychological analgesia in childbirth could be achieved only by joint research carried out by specialists in the various fields concerned. Accordingly, I brought together a team of psychiatrists, psychoanalysts, psychologists, sociologists, psychophysiologists, statisticians, and others, who worked in association with obstetricians at the maternity department of the Hôpital Rothschild, Paris.

When our research team began work, the most widespread method of preparation for childbirth in France was already the psychoprophylactic method (PPM). Its efficacy was widely recognized, although its theoretical foundations remained controversial. The explanations advanced were derived from Pavlovian physiology. They failed, however, to provide any psychological explanation of the role of the interpersonal factor in the operation of the method. The importance of this factor had been clearly evident to me in studies of hypnosis, the interpersonal relationship involved here being capable of producing a sufficient degree of analgesia for childbirth, and even for certain surgical operations. To be sure, the founders of the PPM themselves recognized this function of hypnosis, the hypno-suggestive method (HSM) having served as experimental model in the development of the new method. The PPM had the undeniable advantage of being applicable on a large scale, whereas the HSM required its practitioners to have had more specialized training and remained of limited applicability. But the founders of the PPM had also eliminated the hypnotic relationship because they regarded it as passive, involuntary, and non-conscious. They had replaced it by the pedagogic relationship, which was regarded, on the other hand, as active, voluntary, and fully conscious. This opposition, however, seemed to us too uncompromising and we felt that in both methods the relationship involved unconscious elements, which operated in a concentrated form, as it were, in the hypno-suggestive method, and in a diluted form in the PPM, but in both cases had analgesic effects. With this as a starting-point, our research group oriented its work towards relational or interpersonal psychology.

Our general hypothesis was that pain in childbirth would be related to anxiety-producing factors, themselves dependent upon the woman's whole personality. Since the success or failure of the method depends to a considerable extent upon the woman's personality, it seemed reasonable to suppose that greater understanding of the personality might provide some means of estimating the probable degree of success. For this purpose we used semi-directed interviews and tests, which were given to both prepared and unprepared women. We used semi-directed interviews because this method enabled us to get material of greater depth than that which would have been obtained by direct questioning, and of greater quantity than would have been possible from the study of individual cases. We also collated observations made during the confinements by the professionally trained midwives of the maternity department and by a member of our team, for both prepared and unprepared women, and related these observations to the results of our interviews.

Our work encountered considerable difficulties at the methodological level. In the first place, there is no objective method of measuring pain. Further, we could find no way of classifying the women that was suitable for our research. It was only after many tentative attempts that we developed the tools we needed.

For the measurement of pain, we developed a scale based upon obstetrical, behavioural, and psychological data. In view of the inadequacy of existing typological classifications, we established a scale of 'negativity' intended to provide a personal inventory of all the historical and psychological factors capable of causing anxiety during pregnancy and confinement. These factors are, moreover, those that emerge most clearly by themselves, since, in semi-directed interviews, it is almost always negative aspects that are considered the most important to report. The field of investigation was divided into several areas – body, femininity, family environment, social adjustment, and so on. After completing our work, we were able to demonstrate overall relationships between the negativity index, the degree of preparation, and the painfulness of the confinement. These may subsequently be used by other researchers as a basis for making prognoses about the pain and the course of confinements, and thus for prescribing adequate preparation. Furthermore, we attempted to establish particular relationships for special areas of the negativity inquiry. We hoped thereby to find a more direct means of access to the area of personality most significantly related to confinement, which would give future practitioners a more usable and effective tool.

We make no claim to have solved the delicate problems facing us. We should feel satisfied if our research were to be regarded as a pioneering work, raising many questions and offering empirical grounds for some tentative answers. We hope that the paths of research thus opened will be followed one day by those who have already been engaged in this work or by others who may be interested.

We believe that this book will be of interest to practitioners of obstetrics as well as to research workers. Through study of the psychological aspects of motherhood, they may find that they can adopt an even more understanding attitude to their patients and increase the effectiveness of their work. Again, through the illustrative case-histories that it contains, the book may perhaps allow practitioners to add to their knowledge in this field, thus providing them with additional evidence on which to base their prognoses of their patients' behaviour during confinement. Lastly, by providing a comprehensive and up-to-date survey of the literature, the book will inform any interested readers about recent and current research in this field and its potential contribution to obstetrical psychosomatics.

I must now, on behalf of myself and my co-authors in the present work, acknowledge our debt to our friend, the late Muriel Cahen, for the large part she played in getting our project under way. We further wish to express our gratitude to all those who, at various stages in the research, gave us most valuable assistance: N. Alphandery, M. Chiva, M. Gluge, M. L. Mondzain, and B. This. We are particularly indebted to Roger Perron, who assisted us in the methodological and statistical treatment of our data, and in the interpretation of the results.

We have also to thank most sincerely those who were kind enough to give us their assistance as consultants: Mme J. Favez-Boutonier, Professor of Psychology at the Sorbonne; P. Pichot, Professor of Medical Psychology in the Faculty of Medicine; and M. Vincent-Bloch, lecturer at the Sorbonne.

Our research could not have been carried out without the generous financial support of the Foundations Fund for Research in Psychiatry. My personal contacts with the chairman of the Foundations Board of Directors, F. C. Redlich, Professor of Psychiatry at Yale University, with the treasurer, W. Lippard, Dean of the Faculty of Medicine at Yale, and with the executive officer, M. L. Levin, and his successor Clark Bailey, have always been marked by a high degree of cordiality.

Our thanks are due to the Ligue Française d'Hygiène Mentale, which accorded us its sponsorship, and especially to Professor P. Sivadon, secretary-general of the Ligue until 1961 and a member of its scientific committee, for his continued interest in our work. We also wish to express our gratitude to Dr Bergeron and Professor Deniker, members of the scientific committee, and to Dr C. Veil, the present secretary-general, M E. Breuillard, the treasurer, and Mlle J. Duron, the administrative secretary.

Mme Cariot, our research secretary, gave us most valuable help at all stages of our work.

Finally, we wish to record our deep gratitude to Dr P. Walter, who gave us the benefit of his wide clinical experience, was unstinting of helpful advice, and greatly facilitated our work in his department. The assistance received from the obstetrical staff in this department, especially the midwives, was invaluable.

L.C.

CHAPTER 1

History and Theory of Psychosomatic Methods of Preparation for Childbirth

With the advent of psychosomatic methods of preparation for childbirth – Read's method and the psychoprophylactic method – psychosomatics effectively launched itself into the field of obstetrics. The women who were the subjects of the present investigation were prepared by the psychoprophylactic method. In this chapter, however, the theoretical bases of all the methods will be reviewed so that the reader may get an overall view of the problems which have been the object of such lively controversy (29). We shall first of all give a brief historical account of those experiments in psychological analgesia which were the predecessors of the methods of preparation for childbirth in current use, and then proceed to describe the development of these methods and the theoretical problems to which they give rise.

HISTORICAL REVIEW[1]

THE HYPNO-SUGGESTIVE METHOD

It is difficult to understand the current methods of preparation for childbirth without saying a word about the experiments in psychological analgesia in obstetrics which preceded them. These experiments were based essentially upon hypnosis. They were first tried at the end of the nineteenth century in France and elsewhere, and were resumed after the First World War in Germany and Austria. In Russia, experiments in hypnotic analgesia were begun about 1923 and continued, with interruptions, up to the present time; in the United States, they began in 1943. Nowhere did the experiments lead to mass application; thus in 1954 Velvovski *et al.* (152) estimated the number

---

[1] For a more detailed treatment of the historical aspect, see (28).

1

of published cases of hypnotic analgesia in thirty years in the Soviet Union at 8,000. In the United States, the hypno-suggestive method has been used only on a limited scale.

We need not go into the complex reasons for the failure of hypnotic analgesia to be applied on a large scale. It need only be observed that hypnosis remains surrounded by a kind of magic halo which creates resistance, among doctors as well as among members of the public; and that the practice of hypnosis requires psychotherapeutic training. From a theoretical point of view, nevertheless, these experiments in hypnotic analgesia are of primary importance. They represent macroscopic and peculiarly impressive examples of analgesic effects obtained by psychological means. The material that has been left to us by these early researchers is valuable for the extent to which it casts light upon the problem of the experience of pain. These authors show us, in effect, the complexity of the problem by demonstrating empirically the variety of the 'patterns' of analgesia: the patient may be aware of contractions of the uterus without experiencing the slightest pain; or the pain may be lessened; or again, in spite of the pain, the patient may remain calm, or even say that she is not suffering while at the same time showing all the autonomic signs of pain; or she may even forget the whole thing.

An important phase in the history of psychological analgesia was reached through the work of the Viennese psychiatrist Kogerer (84) about 1922, which can be related to some old experiments of Liébeault (98). Liébeault had used hypnotic analgesia for minor surgical operations in a new way, obtaining the analgesic effect by post-hypnotic suggestion. The operations themselves were performed in the normal state of wakefulness. Kogerer adopted this procedure in the field of obstetrics. Where did he get the idea of doing this? He had been struck by an observation made by von Oettingen of Heidelberg (121). Von Oettingen had remarked that some prepared women were late in arriving at the labour ward, after the rupture of the membranes. They had, in fact, never felt the contractions. One of them had actually given birth without pain in a fully conscious state. Von Oettingen, believing this woman not to have been under hypnosis during labour, felt that he could not count her case as a success. But Kogerer saw the possibility of considerably extending the application of hypnotic analgesia in obstetrics, since it appeared no longer necessary to use hypnosis at the actual time of labour.

2

Theoretically, this discovery introduced a new dimension in hypnotically produced analgesia: the analgesia need not necessarily be the temporal accompaniment of hypnosis, but may be subject to a certain delay effect. Hypnosis being only, as we have stated, a particular kind of exaggerated and intense form of psychotherapeutic relationship, one might expect other forms of this relationship, even non-hypnotic forms, to be capable of producing deferred or contemporaneous analgesia. These other forms of relationship are seen at work in the non-hypnotic methods of obstetrical analgesia.

NATURAL CHILDBIRTH (NC) AND THE PSYCHOPROPHYLACTIC METHOD (PPM)

The earliest stage in the history of psychological analgesia in childbirth was characterized by the use of hypnosis as the analgesic procedure. The methods which were subsequently elaborated and which today are widely applied no longer use hypnosis. These are Read's method (137) and the psychoprophylactic method or PPM (151, 152). The latter, first used in 1949, is a direct outcome of the hypno-suggestive experiments which have just been discussed. The method developed by the English physician, Grantley Dick Read, described in 1933, was the result of a fruitful intuition: confronted with a woman in labour who refused chloroform, saying that she was not in pain, Read had the 'revelation', in his own words, 'that there was no law in nature and no design that could justify the pain of childbirth' (137, p. 6). From this starting-point, Read conceived his method of natural childbirth, the principles of which can be summarized as follows: certain sociocultural factors produce fear, which leads to tension, which, in turn, causes pain (the triad Fear-Tension-Pain). Fear is dissipated by information and education, and tension is removed by relaxation.

The psychoprophylactic method, introduced by Velvovski and his collaborators, started from an experimental basis. For twenty-five years they had been using hypno-suggestive methods, and had come to the following conclusions: pain is not a necessary accompaniment of childbirth; verbal suggestion can have an analgesic effect; finally, fear and anxiety are very important factors in pain during childbirth. These conclusions served as a theoretical basis for the elaboration of a new method which could be applied on a large scale and in which effects could be produced verbally by means other than hypnosis.

3

These psychoprophylactic factors, which indeed played a supporting role in the hypno-suggestive method, for writers like Platonov (128), Shlifer (144a), Kopil-Levina (86), Zdravomyslov (158), etc., consist of information, education, the removal of fear, the creation of positive feeling, good relations between therapist and patient, and a favourable environment in the maternity department. In the PPM, it is hypnosis that now plays the supporting role in difficult cases.

The psychoprophylactic method has developed rapidly and seems to have given new impetus to Read's method, which up to 1950 had met with only limited success. The success and spread of the PPM in France set the fashion, and the French doctors Lamaze (90) and Vellay (149, 150) were mainly responsible for its wide diffusion in Western Europe and South America.

THEORETICAL PROBLEMS

If one considers the principles stated by their authors, the two methods appear theoretically very different from one another. Read attributes to fear the main role in the development of pain and makes the removal of fear the essential condition of analgesia. The Soviet school, while admitting the importance of fear, brings in a whole series of conditioned mechanisms. But when one looks closer, one finds that both these interpretations are hypothetical. The famous triad referred to by Read – Fear-Tension-Pain – no doubt represents a fruitful intuition, but the idea requires to be elaborated and confirmed by physiological observation.

The psychoprophylactic method has been believed, outside the Soviet Union, to rest upon a monolithic explanation. In fact, the various authors are scarcely agreed on any but very general points, such as the role of the cortex in childbirth and in the perception of pain, and the particular importance of the spoken word. Their differences become apparent as soon as we come to the more specific problems, which are more important for a physiological interpretation of the method. Thus, uterine contraction is considered by Velvovski (as also by Read) as physiologically painless, but he is almost the only Soviet author to hold this view. Then again, Velvovski, who to start with viewed all pain during childbirth as a conditioned response, later admitted pains of localized somatic origin and 'functional' pains, the result of 'cerebral' disturbances provoked by fear, unpleasant emotions, beliefs, etc. But these views are likewise contested, the very idea of conditioned pain in childbirth being questioned (Davidenkov, 39).

Other differences are becoming apparent as to the mode of action of the essential factor in the PPM, education. For Velvovski, education produces analgesia in an entirely new way: whereas, in the hypno-suggestive method, analgesia was achieved by 'cortical inhibition' and involved a *therapeutic* process, according to Velvovski it is achieved in the PPM by 'activation', through raising of the cortical threshold for pain. The process is *prophylactic*, it aims at *preventing* pain and no longer at *suppressing* it. Here again, there are but few Soviet authors who follow Velvovski, and some (e.g. Doline and Salgannik, 46, 143) even hold that, when there is analgesia in the PPM, it is always the result of a process of inhibition. For our part we would point out that the distinction between analgesia brought about by inhibition and analgesia resulting from activation has as yet no experimentally demonstrated basis.

The progress of electrophysiological investigation of the central nervous system has shown that inhibitory mechanisms are involved in 'directional' or oriented attention in animals. It has been demonstrated that, if a particularly meaningful stimulus is presented to an animal, there is inhibition of the transmission of information from other sensory modalities. The location of these inhibitory mechanisms, however, is still largely unsettled (Hernandez-Peon, Scherrer, and Jouvet, 69; Worden and Marsh, 157). Similarly, certain mechanisms of attention in man have been investigated neurophysiologically (Jouvet, 80). Now if the stimulus, instead of being limited to sensory impression, consists of a verbal or infra-verbal communication, its 'significance' is enriched by an affective charge which considerably increases its inhibitory power, in a manner which varies as a function of the personality of the subject and his relations with the operator. It is precisely a situation of this kind that is involved in suggestion.

A whole book could be written on the problem of suggestion. Here, it will suffice merely to indicate that the role of suggestion in the PPM is variously regarded by Soviet writers. In contrast to Velvovski, who regards it as negligible, some authors, such as Konstantinov (85), assign to it the principal role. We shall return to this problem when we examine in detail the factors involved in the method (p. 16 below).

5

Another difficult theoretical problem is the question of 'nervous types'. Pavlov (125), renewing the Hippocratic tradition, established a fourfold classification for animals. He distinguished the following types:

well-balanced, calm type (phlegmatic)
well-balanced, lively type (sanguine)
strong excitatory type (choleric)
weak inhibitory type (melancholic).

How far must we take account of the nervous type in the application of the PPM? For Velvovski (151) this plays no part in childbirth, except in pathological cases. Other writers assign to it some importance. All agree that it is difficult to determine the nervous type, for this requires the consideration of a large number of parameters: the strength, the lability, and the nature of the relations between activation and inhibition; and certain peculiarities in the relations between the first and second signalling systems, and between the cortex and the sub-cortical region. The methods used are more or less elaborate: they depend on tests (e.g. tests of suggestibility, the word association test) and on anamnestic data. Some writers talk of particular typological characteristics, others of 'emotional predispositions'. In other words, these methods are the kind of thing that we would call a psychological investigation of personality. Thus, in an anamnesis used by Plotitcher (130) to determine nervous type, inquiries are made about the relations of the expectant mother with her parents, her husband, her children, her relatives, and her social environment, about her professional activity, about her ability to adapt to new tasks, etc.

The difficulties experienced by Soviet writers in determining nervous type arise essentially from the fact that the classification, based initially on animals, cannot be transposed unmodified to man. In man, the social takes precedence over the biological. This is why certain words can exert an effect on one individual and have no effect on another; for the response depends upon past experience. It should be added that interpersonal relations are not necessarily established only on the verbal level, and that there is a level of emotional relationship in which speech is not necessarily involved. As Ajuriaguerra (3) has pointed out, a deaf mute can no doubt be effectively prepared for childbirth just like a normal woman. In short, the direct methods of investigation used by the Russian writers do not seem to be sufficient to reveal

6

adequately the past experience of the individual. For this past experience includes both conscious and unconscious components and it is difficult to reach the latter by means of direct questioning. We must, of course, recognize that methods using modern psychoanalytic concepts with a view to laying bare the deep levels of the personality are still in course of development, as will emerge more clearly later, when the present research is described.

These controversies have not had much place in the theoretical writings of French adherents of the PPM. For some time they have used the terminology of Pavlovian physiology (4, 153), adopting mainly the ideas of Velvovski. In 1956, one of the present writers (27) expressed certain reservations about the explanatory value of ideas derived exclusively from Pavlovian physiology, and has since insisted upon the need to study psychological and interpersonal aspects. This point of view seems to have gained ground.[1] A change began to appear in 1959. It was admitted that the first theoretical expositions of the method were, in the words actually used by one of them, 'rough and narrowly conceived' (109). New points of view were expressed. Vermorel (154) abandoned the use of Pavlovian terminology to 'translate' psychological phenomena, and resorted to a form of expression which included a number of concepts in their psychoanalytic sense – anxiety, unconscious motives, fantasies, orality, transference, etc. He made frequent reference to authors such as Helene Deutsch (44) and Gressot (66). For him, the PPM is above all a form of education, although he explicitly states, 'it is its psychotherapeutic effects with which we are concerned'. This refers, of course, to a superficial kind of psychotherapy, limited to pregnancy and confinement.

Angelergues (5) favours 'the perfectly legitimate rejection of Pavlovian ideas in psychology and psychopathology'. He does not, however, turn to the concepts of interpersonal dynamic psychology to replace them. He admits that Pavlovian ideas are still valuable in relation to training, which is for him the basis of the PPM. He believes that there is some 'accidental and fortuitous' psychotherapy in all training, but considers that it is negligible, holding that true psychotherapy is that which effects structural changes in the personality. Training, he says, 'has as its aim the adjustment of the woman to a

[1] This theoretical development can also be observed in a fairly recent issue of the *Bull. Soc. internat. de Psychoprophylaxie obstétricale*, 6, 1964, which includes a series of articles dealing mainly with interpersonal relations.

specific situation, and can attain this end only in so far as this situation is experienced as an event relatively isolated from her personality as a whole. In preparing the woman, we aim to provide her with a weapon against her own personality, by using the processes of conditioning.'

Another French writer, Muldworf, is one of those who seem most attached to the explanatory value of Pavlovian physiology for the method. His views are expressed in three papers (109, 110, 111) read at the three successive congresses of the Société française de Psychoprophylaxie obstétricale in 1959, 1960, and 1961. He agrees that we must 'transcend the physiological narrowness of misinterpreted Pavlovism', but immediately adds that 'Pavlovian experimentation is still the basis on which the theory of psychoprophylaxis is erected' (110). Since the physiology of conditioning is 'a very complex experimental entity', 'beyond our scope', Muldworf abandons any attempt to explain pain during labour and psychological analgesia on the basis of the formation or extinction of conditioned reflexes. 'This', he says, 'would be an illegitimate and anti-scientific transposition from one field – physiology – to another, psychology' (111).

He, too, wants to see psychoprophylaxis above all as a form of instruction, this term including both education and training. He considers that there is at present no psychological theory that takes due account of instruction, and he criticizes psychoanalysis in particular. There remains rational, common-sense psychology, which persuades and informs, helps the woman to resolve her present conflicts, guides her towards the solution of her difficulties, reduces her negative feelings, and so on.

On the problem of the nature of pain during labour, Muldworf (109) maintains a position close to that of Velvovski. He considers that childbirth is normally painless, and that pain is the result of psychological and sociocultural factors. Thus the effects of the method would be at a prophylactic level.

The controversies among Soviet writers, and the various points of view among French writers, confirm that the P P M has not yet acquired any sound theoretical basis. The relations between psychoprophylaxis and psychotherapy are not made clear. One is reminded here of the discussion between Bernheim and Dubois of Berne at the beginning of the century, the one using suggestion and the other persuasion, the former identifying the two ideas, while the latter strongly emphasized their differences. As far as analgesia is concerned, we have experimental evidence that it can be achieved by suggestion, whereas the analgesic effectiveness of persuasion remains to be demonstrated.

A similar problem arises concerning the analgesic effect of instruction. We have already noted the importance attached to instruction by French writers. Indeed, they use three different terms – instruction, education, and training – without always distinguishing clearly between them. They recognize the psychotherapeutic value of instruction, but do not indicate the respective parts played by the intellectual aspects, the affective aspects, and the motor aspects of which it is made up. If mere knowledge by itself does not appear to have any direct analgesic effect, the affective aspect, introducing an interpersonal element, opens the way to experimentally demonstrated analgesia. At a different level, a degree of analgesia can be achieved by using 'pain-preventing procedures' based on 'cortical activity' or distraction of attention, previously also known as indirect suggestion.

One can hold that all instruction, all training, every acquisition or enrichment of the ego (whether it involves learning a foreign language or learning to ski) modifies to a certain degree the deeper layers of the personality of the person concerned, with eventual repercussions on sensitivity to pain. But this is only a hypothesis for which it would be difficult to find experimental support, in view of the numerous links in the chain between cause and supposed effect.

The point of view of Angelergues, who would enclose the pregnant woman in her own special state, disregarding her personal drama, by representing childbirth to her as a job of work, a particular task to accomplish, requiring an *active*, conscious mental attitude, calls for some comment. First of all, is such an attitude sufficient to effect analgesia, in view of the fact that pain in childbirth is influenced by the deeper levels of the personality? Second, if analgesia is achieved, is it not in large part due to suggestion, to the 'exhortations' of the person undertaking the preparation? Finally, if it is desirable for the woman to be active and to cooperate, it is also necessary to ensure that her activity is not pushed too far, and does not encourage a masculine protest reaction. For then the very activity which, according to Angelergues, should prevent the woman from becoming neurotic would paradoxically end in making her so.

Is the psychotherapy in psychoprophylactic instruction genuine psychotherapy? The answers given by the writers considered are

9

reserved and ambiguous. Vermorel agrees that in the PPM, as in all psychotherapy, there are emotional exchanges. 'The doctor or midwife', he says, 'plays a role analogous to that of the parents towards the young child.' But he equally asserts that 'the psychoprophylactic method is not, properly speaking, psychotherapy in the strict sense of the term; it is rather a kind of instruction, with secondary psychotherapeutic effects' (154). For Muldworf (111), 'psychoprophylaxis is a form of training, not of psychotherapy. It is a kind of instruction with psychotherapeutic aims and effects, but it is not a form of psychotherapy in the proper sense of the term.' Angelergues, as we have seen, refuses to place psychoprophylaxis among the psychotherapies.

It seems to us that the woman who receives instruction, theoretical and practical, *with a view to painless childbirth*, at once puts herself in a psychotherapeutic situation. It is true that this does not imply deep psychotherapy, as Angelergues emphasizes, but this is not sufficient reason for refusing, as he does, to allow it the very name of psychotherapy. The PPM may not be concerned with psychotherapy that includes insight, interpretation, etc., but the woman nevertheless finds herself in a network of relationships, and psychodynamic forces are aroused.[1] It might be viewed as a kind of short psychotherapy, superficial, gratifying, invigorating, and so on. It often yields speedy positive results, for pregnant women are particularly receptive. In fact, pregnancy provokes an emotional 'crisis' (14, 15) in all women, and they appear more neurotic than they really are. Brief and superficial psychotherapy may then be effective. But it seems to us that this can be effectively given by the obstetrician, who thus remains 'the central and directing person', as Angelergues requires (5). It is true that it is desirable for him to take an interest in the psychological aspects of his relations with the future mother, but this is something to be found in every act of medical practice. On this point he will find an adviser in the person of the psychiatrist attached to his unit. The role of the psychiatrist will be more important in cases with clear psychopathology requiring specialized psychotherapeutic care.

The problem of the relationship between psychiatrists and other practitioners arises, furthermore, in other fields of medicine. The

[1] Valabrega, in his book *La relation thérapeutique* (148), emphasizes the markedly psychotherapeutic character of the relationships of the woman to the obstetrician and to the person concerned with her preparation (cf. p. 264 below).

doctor treating the case remains the person principally involved and, as Balint (7) has noted, he is in the best position to deal with the emotional aspects of the patient.

These controversies received a new impetus at the congress of the Société française de Psychoprophylaxie obstétricale held at Strasbourg in May 1963 (23), where they centred on the theme 'psychoanalysis and psychoprophylaxis' or 'depth psychology and surface psychology' (see Appendix II). The heat generated on both sides indicates what a delicate matter it is to attempt, in our present state of knowledge and with our present tools of investigation, to delimit psychotherapy and psychoprophylaxis in psychological analgesia in obstetrics.

FACTORS INVOLVED IN THE METHODS

If we now compare the methods of Read and Velvovski on the practical level, we cannot fail to be struck by their similarities, in spite of their differences in origin and in theoretical interpretation. Both actually include the same didactic and psychotherapeutic factors: instruction in the anatomical and physiological facts of childbirth, removal of fear, creation of positive feelings, a good relationship between the staff involved in preparation and the expectant mother, and a good emotional atmosphere in the labour ward.

The only differences have to do with physiotherapeutic factors (here we include relaxation, breathing, and physical exercises) (cf. 29). Given the importance of the educational and especially the psychotherapeutic factors, which are the same in both methods, these differences, which, as will presently be shown, are small, cannot mask the very great similarity between Read's method and Velvovski's.

Let us now consider more closely the operation of the factors we have just enumerated, examining the part played by each of them in achieving the various kinds of advantages accruing from the method. At the end of the chapter (pp. 18-19) the reader will find three deliberately simplified schematic tables indicating the possible modes of operation of these factors.

EDUCATIONAL FACTOR

The instruction given may not, perhaps, directly bring analgesia, for knowledge of the anatomical-physiological mechanism of childbirth does not prevent midwives or women doctors from experiencing pain. No doubt it may be thought that, since it eliminates ignorance and the fear that results from it, the educational factor contributes indirectly to the analgesia. But there is no experimental evidence on this point. In any case, even if there is no analgesic effect, the elimination of ignorance is psychologically beneficial to the woman. In psychoanalytic terms, it might be said that it replaces fantasies by facts, as emphasized by Donovan and Landisberg (50), although only partly, since not all fantasies can be exorcised by facts alone.

Education is equally important on the social level, by raising the standard of knowledge, and on the individual level, by enabling the expectant mother to enrich her personality and thereby to strengthen her ego. Moreover, it is via the educational factor that the woman establishes interpersonal relations with the obstetrician and the members of his team. But we are now touching on the question of interpersonal relations, to which we shall return in connexion with the psychotherapeutic factor.

PHYSIOTHERAPEUTIC FACTOR

Under this heading are included physical exercises, breathing exercises, and relaxation.

The practice of *physical exercises* is useful in improving the general physical and mental tone. As far as effects on analgesia are concerned, opinions are divided. Some writers think that such exercises have a beneficial effect on the outcome of the pregnancy, others hold that athletic and very muscular women have more painful confinements. Physical exercises form part of Read's method, and have been developed particularly in Germany and German-speaking Switzerland. They constituted no part of the psychoprophylactic method at the beginning, but some Soviet writers, such as Nicolaiev (117), advocate them at the present time. In France, the most orthodox practitioners of the PPM do not use them.

Breathing exercises (during pregnancy and confinement) are recommended by all the methods. They are used, with various rhythms, by Read and his followers, but their mode of action is not clearly explained. Sometimes they are said to contribute to the maintenance of the general tone of the woman, sometimes to increase the supply of oxygen to the uterus during labour, sometimes to facilitate general relaxation. A rapid breathing rhythm, described in a work by Read which appeared in 1955 and was reissued in 1957, is claimed to be of great value in labour, during contractions (138, p. 22).

The German writer Prill (131), a follower of Read, attaches especial importance to the regularity of the respiratory rhythm (not only for childbirth, incidentally, but for all human activity).

The Soviet writers teach their expectant mothers a deep-breathing rhythm to be practised, later, during contractions. They regard it as a 'pain-killing' procedure because it creates, in Pavlovian terms, a focus of cortical activation, in other words, a distraction of attention.

The Lamaze school has introduced a new kind of breathing during dilatation – 'rapid, superficial breathing'; its aim, according to some, is to increase the supply of oxygen, and, according to others, to effect a 'concentration upon cortical activity' (which amounts to a distraction of attention). This latter effect is undeniable. But the supply of oxygen is a different matter. It is possible that rapid respiration, on the contrary, produces a hypercapnia which, by bringing about a rise in the threshold of awareness, may have an analgesic effect. It should be noted that panting of this kind has never been used in the Soviet Union. Nicolaiev, writing in 1964 (120), comments as follows: 'Panting should be discouraged, since the hyperpnoea provokes twilight states.' It may also be mentioned that in France the use of panting is limited; it is employed only for a very short period of time, and is replaced during the greater part of labour by deep breathing with vigorous exhalation.

It appears, then, that the connexion between breathing exercises and analgesia properly speaking is still not well understood and may exist at several levels. The Yogis, who can achieve complete anaesthesia, use breathing exercises to put themselves into a state of 'trance'. Finally, it must not be forgotten that respiration is closely connected with the emotional life. Thus the sigh corresponds to a state of 'feeling', and fear and anger are both bound up with modifications of the respiratory rhythm.

We now come to what is perhaps the most controversial problem, that of *relaxation*. We should not be surprised that this is so. By its double physical and mental aspect, relaxation raises difficulties which are inherent in psychosomatics and are encountered whenever the relations between physiology and psychology are investigated. The idea of relaxation occurs in all the methods, whether it is expressed by this term, or by the words 'relaxing rest', as with Soviet writers, or

13

by the term 'controlled relaxation', as in the PPM as practised in France. But it appears in various guises and is interpreted in various ways. The position is confused. For Read, relaxation plays an especially important role, since it has to get rid of tension, which constitutes one of the elements of the famous triad. Read and his adherents claim to derive their practice from the 'progressive relaxation' of Jacobson (74), although Jacobson himself denies the similarity (75).

For Helen Heardman (68), one of Read's followers, there are two forms of relaxation, one 'mental', which occurs when the mind is at rest, and the other 'physical' or 'conscious', which is accompanied by intense mental concentration. The latter, regarded as the more important, is practised during advanced dilatation. It is used sparingly, since – and this may appear paradoxical – it is fatiguing. It is, then, an 'activity': we might say, in Pavlovian terms, that it is a 'concentration on cortical activity', thus equivalent to a 'pain-killing procedure' and analogous to respiration. But this relaxation is not always 'active', since Read himself has observed that it may lead to states approaching unconsciousness with amnesia. This last aspect has not escaped the American writers who use the hypno-suggestive methods, such as Kroger (88, 89) and Abramson and Heron (2). They consider that relaxation includes hypno-suggestive elements and that it is equivalent to a mild hypnotic state, with increased suggestibility. We now reach a new dimension, and relaxation appears in relation to a factor on another level, the interpersonal factor.

The Soviet writers, moreover, join the American critics in holding that Read's relaxation is a hypno-suggestive procedure, inaugurated in Russia thirty-five years ago and still used to a limited extent, although not part of the psychoprophylactic method, except in difficult cases. Nicolaiev (120), indeed, observes that relaxation may have the undesirable effect of raising the threshold of awareness and thus impeding the application of the PPM. Now, the Soviet writers claim to have abandoned hypno-suggestive methods because they cannot be applied on a large scale. But if they regard Read's method as being hypno-suggestive, how do they account for the fact that it *does* lend itself to large-scale application? Again, if they recognize the role of suggestion in relaxation, they ignore its intersubjective psychological aspect. For them, relaxation is accompanied by hypnoidal states during which one can, by verbal methods, extinguish harmful reflexes and establish beneficial ones. These hypnoidal states were used in the PPM itself in its early days, to 'consolidate' instruction and 'pain-killing procedures'. They were abandoned about 1953–54.

The Lamaze school practises a form of relaxation similar to Read's, but gives it a different theoretical interpretation, concentrating largely on its active aspect. Lamaze was probably inspired by the 'relaxing rest' technique which he had seen in practice in the USSR in 1951, at the time when it was still used with all women prepared by the PPM. He does not seem to have suspected that the procedure was meant to have a suggestive effect. Thus the idea of relaxation is enveloped in misunderstandings.

How have these misunderstandings arisen? What explanation can there be for the fact that, for some, relaxation is an active phenomenon, for others passive; that for some it is accompanied by suggestion and for others it is not? We can, perhaps, answer these questions by saying that relaxation is a complex phenomenon with more than one aspect, and that the different authors, according to their theoretical predispositions, have favoured this or that aspect at the expense of others (30). Relaxation operates on several levels between the two poles of the physiological and the psychological; and these levels are not clearly delimited, but more or less overlapping. For convenience in exposition, relaxation can be assigned, schematically, three levels of action:

the muscular level
the central level (attention)
the psychotherapeutic level (interpersonal experience and suggestion).

At the muscular level, relaxation undoubtedly reduces tension. But instruments for measuring this are still imperfect; and it has not been demonstrated experimentally that relaxation is accompanied by analgesia.

At the central or neurophysiological level, relaxation involves the well-known phenomenon of attention. It is empirically established that stimulation which is the object of attention tends to eclipse other contemporaneous stimulation. There is an 'active' mechanism of concentration, distraction, or diversion, or, in Pavlovian language, of concentration on a focus of cortical activation. This mechanism is beginning to be investigated, as we have said, by modern electrophysiological techniques applied to animals and even to man. But it would be naïve to regard this simply as the quantitative, neurophysiological aspect of attention. As the American writer Rapaport (136) has emphasized, the mechanism by which the perception of pain is modified does not consist of 'a certain amount of attention shifted from one place to another'; it is 'a matter of complex dynamics and not a simple shift of quantity. We deal here with qualitative changes and multiple dimensions.' The emotional significance of the stimulus is important. Attempts have been made to relate the idea of attention to that of transference in the psychoanalytic sense. Thus Margaret Brenman (19) has said of women who have given birth under hypnosis: 'Attention, if we can use that undefined concept here, was directed to whatever the physician was doing and was so "gratifying" that possibly the experience of pain was not so important any longer.' It can therefore be seen that attention may be directed, not only to the relaxing activity itself, but to the person of the 'relaxer'. This brings us to the third level, that of psychotherapeutic action proper.

Relaxation permits the establishment of an interpersonal relationship between the subject and the person who is preparing her, with all the immediate or deferred psychotherapeutic consequences thereof. This is the 'passive' aspect of relaxation.

It may be asked to what extent the three levels of operation of relaxation act together. It seems to us that it is, above all, the personality of the woman and her psycho-affective development that determine this. Every woman will make relaxation a more or less profitable experience, whether passive or active. Some women will, as it were, operate on the interpersonal level, and analgesia will be obtained through emotional channels. Others will use relaxation in a more 'mechanical' way, concentrating their attention upon some activity. And others still may profit from these two aspects, using the first during preparation and the second during confinement. But we must not lose sight of the importance of the personality of the individual who is undertaking the preparation, and of the type of relationship he establishes with the expectant mother.

These intrapersonal and interpersonal problems bring us directly to the psychotherapeutic factor, which we shall now examine.

PSYCHOTHERAPEUTIC FACTOR

All the writers we have cited admit the central role of the psychotherapeutic factor in the application of the methods. Although it is

16

here considered separately for the purposes of exposition, this factor is involved in all the constituents of the methods, in so far as there is contact between two or more persons. Read insists on the necessity of a good atmosphere in preparation, on the importance of building up the woman's confidence, and on the suggestive power of the doctor. Velvovski, who prefers the term psychoprophylaxis to the term psychotherapy, lays just as much stress on a good atmosphere during preparation and in the labour ward, and on the attentive and benevolent attitude required of the doctor. Preparation carried out unfeelingly and without enthusiasm, he says, is doomed to failure. We ourselves have observed that a well-prepared woman, if she is left alone during confinement, does not generally achieve complete success.

What, then, is the nature of the psychotherapeutic factor? Reference has already been made to the many controversies on the question of whether it can be reduced to suggestion or not. In fact, there is established between the woman, the doctor, and the preparation team, a complex of relationships with all their conscious and unconscious motivational ramifications. Suggestion is one form of such relationships. The type of motivation to which it corresponds has never been accurately described, but it is currently associated with submissiveness, absence of a critical attitude, etc. – and hence the pejorative connotation of the term suggestion. But it is our contention that the psychotherapeutic relationship can involve other and more complex types of psychodynamic force. Suggestive analgesia is an empirical fact and it acts directly on pain. But we may suppose that other factors are also conducive to analgesia, in an indirect way, acting at the level of anxiety. At this level, analgesia may be achieved by two mechanisms: in the first, the removal of anxiety directly modifies the perception of pain; in the second, the disappearance of anxiety affects the quality of the uterine contractions (lessening of spasms) and reduces or abolishes the pain by acting on its psychosomatic causes. The hypothesis that anxiety causes pain is here assumed. But things are not as simple as this, for the relations between anxiety and pain are complex. Anxiety works its way into a system of defences within the personality and, at a very deep level, can reduce the pain of childbirth by a denial mechanism. Thus we sometimes see very neurotic women having painless confinements.

The beneficial effects of psychotherapy are not, of course, restricted to analgesia. They are also reflected in the woman's behaviour, in her

17

3

mental equilibrium, and, through psychosomatic correlates, in the physiological quality of the pregnancy and confinement.

Now, the question that arises is: 'Why does a woman choose this or that form of relationship?' We may perhaps answer that the choice that is made is a function of her deeper personality. The study of this deeper personality should therefore bring some measure of increased understanding. The Soviet writers have attempted such a study on the basis of Pavlovian typology, and we have seen the difficulties with which they meet. We have tried to adopt a psychodynamic frame of reference, but very difficult methodological problems are involved.

Chapter 2 outlines the perspectives that psychoanalytic theories have opened for obstetrics, and considers their contribution to the study of the psychology of womanhood, pregnancy, and motherhood.

Tables 1, *2*, and *3* illustrate the significance and the ordering of the different factors in the three methods of analgesia: the hypno-suggestive method, natural childbirth, and the psychoprophylactic method. In the first table, the methods of analgesia are classified according to the importance given to *suggestion* in their mode of action.

TABLE 1   FACTORS RELEVANT TO ANALGESIA AND SUGGESTION

Suggestive factors		Non-suggestive factors	
Suggestive psychotherapy	Pain-reducing procedures	Non-suggestive psychotherapy	Enrichment of the ego
Direct verbal suggestion within the relationship: direct action on the perception of pain	Indirect suggestion by distraction of attention (concentration on cortical activity): breathing, effleurage, massage	Psychodynamic modifications occurring within the relationship: (a) direct action on the perception of pain; (b) effects on the physiological processes involved in pain by action aimed at anxiety	Acquisition of theoretical and technical knowledge: possible repercussions on the perception of pain

Analgesia

TABLE 2   FACTORS RELEVANT TO ANALGESIA AND
INTERPERSONAL RELATIONSHIP

Interpersonal factors		Non-interpersonal factors	
Suggestive psychotherapy	*Non-suggestive psychotherapy*	*Pain-reducing procedures*	*Enrichment of the ego*
Direct verbal suggestion within the relationship: direct action on the perception of pain	Psychodynamic modifications occurring within the relationship: (a) direct action on the perception of pain: (b) effects on the physiological processes involved in pain by action aimed at anxiety	Indirect suggestion by distraction of attention (concentration on cortical activity): breathing, effleurage, massage	Acquisition of theoretical and technical knowledge: possible repercussions on the perception of pain

Analgesia

TABLE 3   INTERPERSONAL AND SUGGESTIVE FACTORS
IN METHODS OF ANALGESIA

Interpersonal factors →

Non-suggestive psychotherapy	*Suggestive psychotherapy*
Psychodynamic modifications occurring within the relationship: (a) direct action on the perception of pain; (b) effects on the physiological processes involved in pain by action directed against anxiety	Direct verbal suggestion within the relationship: direct action on the perception of pain
Enrichment of the ego Acquisition of theoretical and technical knowledge: possible repercussions on the perception of pain	*Pain-reducing procedures* Indirect suggestion by distraction of attention (concentration on cortical activity): breathing, effleurage, massage

Suggestion

In the second, the same methods are classified according to the importance given to the *interpersonal relationship*.

The third table combines the other two. It presents the methods of analgesia in terms of both *interpersonal* and *suggestive factors*. These two factors are represented by two orthogonal axes. Each method of analgesia depends increasingly on one or the other of the two factors, the further it lies from the origin (towards the top of the table for the interpersonal factor, towards the right for the factor of suggestion). Thus, suggestive psychotherapy is of all the methods of analgesia the one that depends principally upon both the interpersonal factor and the factor of suggestion.

These distinctions between factors are introduced to clarify theorization and should be viewed in a purely operational perspective. It is not implied that the opposition between 'suggestive' and 'non-suggestive' on the one hand, and between 'interpersonal' and 'non-interpersonal' on the other hand, should be regarded as absolute. It is clear, for example, that there is an interpersonal variable in the 'pain-reducing procedures' and in the 'enrichment of the ego'; but here it is not the basic factor in effecting analgesia, as it is in the psychotherapeutic methods.

SUMMARY

Childbirth involves biological, psychological, and social factors and is a psychosomatic process *par excellence*. The modern methods of preparation for childbirth – Read's method and the psychoprophylactic method – should therefore be examined and interpreted from a psychosomatic point of view. The first of these methods appeared about 1933 as a result of a fruitful intuition based upon many years of obstetrical practice; the second emerged about 1949 as a development from hypno-suggestive experiments in obstetrical analgesia.

The theoretical bases of the two methods appear different and, indeed, have not yet been conclusively established, as heated controversies concerning their psychoprophylactic or psychotherapeutic effects bear witness.

The ways in which the two methods are used, however, are similar, and both include educational, physiotherapeutic, and psychotherapeutic factors. The relative importance of the three kinds of factor has been variously evaluated. The interpersonal factor would appear to play the most important part, although the roles of the other two should not be minimized. In fact, the results achieved depend to a large extent on the woman's personality and, in particular, on the kinds of interpersonal relationship she establishes with those who are preparing her and with the hospital staff in general. This is the justification for the present research, the aim of which is to investigate the relationships between personality, psychosomatics, and motherhood.

CHAPTER 2

Psychoanalytical Perspectives and Obstetrics

In general, it is not easy to make use of psychoanalytic findings when approaching a field in which they have not previously been employed: there is a serious risk of oversimplifying psychoanalytic concepts in attempting to apply them to a new area of research. This danger is particularly great in the case of obstetrics, in which emotional aspects are of prime significance, because such a field is highly susceptible to psychoanalytic interpretations, which may, as a result, give the impression of being superimposed and of bearing little relation to everyday clinical experience. A specialized research such as ours cannot, however, at the present time, neglect the degree of understanding provided by psychoanalysis. Our immediate problem is therefore to explain which psychoanalytic findings and concepts are relevant to a study focused on childbirth.

To prevent misunderstandings, it should be remembered that the most valuable psychoanalytic data are those gathered during the treatment of women who have found themselves pregnant in the course of their cure. This method provides the best means of estimating the practical importance of fantasy in determining what have been the deeply felt experiences of expectant mothers. Treatment also reveals the precise meaning of dreams, fears, and neurotic symptoms that appear during this period.

But the knowledge acquired in such conditions affects current clinical understanding. The latter leans upon hypotheses, and attributes meanings and causal relationships quite often without being able to justify them in any particular case. Psychoanalytic thinking is reflected in the clinician's attitude, influencing his point of view and extending his means of understanding. There are, of course, dangers, which should not be underestimated. There is a risk in accepting what may appear as a closed system of explanation; and again, the system itself is not established beyond dispute, as the differences of opinion between psychoanalysts indicate.

Psychoanalysis does, however, provide some generally accepted ideas:

(a) the existence of the unconscious, i.e. of a psychic system independent of the conscious system and exercising a determining influence on behaviour;

(b) the importance of referring to ontogenetic development and especially to the first years of life; this development is characterized by the existence of infantile sexuality, i.e. of erotic drives, the release of which produces pleasure; their progressive and conflicting development finally leads to the truly genital stage.

This having been said, we may now proceed to give a brief account of the psychoanalytic view of motherhood in its widest sense, of the psychological and dynamic aspects of pregnancy, and, finally, of confinement. The question with which we are concerned is how far the importance attributed to confinement – for in obstetrics, as in methods of preparation, confinement is very naturally isolated and emphasized – can be justified psychologically, and within which theoretical and practical framework.

MOTHERHOOD

All psychoanalytic writers such as Freud (62), Jones (76, 77, 78), Lampl-de Groot (91, 92), Melanie Klein (82), Karen Horney (72, 73), Benedek (10, 11), Helene Deutsch (43, 44, 45), Marie Bonaparte (16, 17), Racamier (132, 133, 134), Chasseguet-Smirgel (26a), and others, agree in placing motherhood at the centre of woman's psycho-emotional development; in fact, Helene Deutsch writes that a girl becomes a woman in the full sense of the word only when she becomes a mother. The reasons for this general agreement are perhaps not so obvious as might be thought. It may be sufficient to point out that psychoanalysis has, in fact, only taken up the traditional Judaeo-Christian values by which we live and which directly affirm the importance of motherhood. We shall consider later the question of the cultural relativity of such a value.

Formally, motherhood is described as an 'integrative stage' in the woman's life (134, p. 527), the favourable outcome of which is expressed by integration, at the highest possible level, of instinctual drives and ego potential. Maternity is the mark of a *progressive* development

23

culminating in a mother-child relationship. This relationship, which will bring new problems (for the child has to grow up), is viewed here as an end in itself and a source of satisfaction: to have a child, or, rather, to create a child, to give him birth. But this progressive development that takes place with motherhood can come about only as a result of a crisis. This convenient idea, particularly emphasized by Bibring *et al.* (14, 15), indicates that the process of integration necessarily reactivates the woman's past history, with its inevitable conflicts, and raises the question of her identity (Erikson, 52). Thus, motherhood activates powerful and labile psychic processes comparable with those of adolescence; and these must not be assessed clinically with reference to classical semiology. As Bibring points out, the mental state involved normally comes close to a reversible pathological state (13). Such psychic systems are particularly sensitive to *current* environmental factors and conditions of living. As Racamier remarks, 'reactions may be either beneficial or harmful' (134, p. 534). This explains the surprising effectiveness of simple forms of psychotherapy and should not be overlooked in evaluating the importance of the psychotherapeutic aspect of preparation, as indicated in Chapter 1.

Thus, the crisis of maternity – more or less severe or masked – is the lot of every woman, and as such can be regarded, at least in some measure, as general rather than specific to any given case and therefore independent of personal problems.

Some authors, such as Bibring *et al.* (14, 15), appear to think that there is no meaningful connexion between the form of the crisis and the previous personality of the woman. This seems to us a somewhat extreme view, even though such a relationship may be hard to demonstrate. What is experienced during the crisis is a function of the woman's life-history. But these factors are apparent as much in processes of adjustment and in ego defence mechanisms as in libidinal patterns and in the introjected imagos which may come to the surface. The crisis is marked by an unstable equilibrium in the impulse-defence balance, since what is reactivated derives as much from infantile desires as from their mechanisms of control. Thus, if motherhood is progressive, it is also essentially *regressive*. There is, as Freud thought, a rapid reactivation of all the stages of development of the libido.

This is why an attempt can be made to get beyond personal historical events and to recall the course of the woman's psychosexual

24

development with everything it implies, for psychoanalysis, in the way of structuring conflicts. A linear description of such development would not reflect the degree to which unknown and obscure factors still influence the development of womanhood. We shall limit ourselves to indicating, in a very schematic manner, the main problems that are likely to recur during the first experience of motherhood.

The crucial point in the psychosexual development of both sexes is the so-called Oedipus stage (from about five to six years of age), during which the child has contrasting relationships with each of his two parents: his (or her) attraction to the one parent is accompanied by a desire to take the place of the other and to identify with him (or her). In the positive Oedipus situation, the attachment to the parent of the opposite sex is accompanied by an identification with the parent of the same sex. In the negative Oedipus situation, the reverse is the case. The oscillation between these two coexisting situations accounts for the ambivalence that characterizes the child's relationship to each parent. The attainment by the child of outside social interests, especially at school, is bound up with his emergence from the Oedipus situation, from its conflicts and fantasies; and this emergence is made possible by physical maturation, which takes the child into the latency period and is normally accompanied by a repression of his drives. The resolution of the Oedipus complex is associated, for the boy, with the real or imaginary threat to his penis represented by his sexual desires. Parental prohibitions are 'introjected', i.e. internalized in the form of a 'superego' which constitutes the rudiments of a moral conscience and a value system.

Freud's first observations (59) on little girls develop the ideas of Abraham (1) and emphasize that, for the girl, the lack of a penis makes castration not a possible threat but a bitter reality. Two consequences follow: penis envy; and a less urgent need to escape from the Oedipus situation and to develop an uncompromising superego.

Briefly, what this amounts to is that the little girl remains more willingly attached to her father than does the little boy to his mother, in so far as the father, possessing the penis which she lacks, can give her its equivalent in the form of a baby, and this has compensatory value, 'since only women have babies'. This almost universal fantasy of being given a baby by the father remains unconsciously active up to the first pregnancy, which thus has the double function of fulfilling an infantile desire and resolving the initial inadequacy. Freud also

25

draws attention (57) to the prevalence, in the woman's relationship to the man, of the desire to *be loved*, the progression to a less narcissistic relationship being effected only through the child who becomes an object of her love.

But let us examine the position a little closer. If these fantasies of the little girl are as important as psychoanalysis considers them to be, this is because they are sources of pleasure, because they are connected with the pleasure of masturbation. At this level, a parallel can be drawn between the development of the little girl and that of the little boy (since the clitoris, which is the main erogenous zone during the Oedipus phase, is the equivalent of a small penis). In so far as the pleasure that it provides is depreciated by the perception of its intrinsic inferiority, the problem arises as to how the erotic sensitivity can be transferred to the vagina. This is an uncertain and complex process, as is shown by the frequency of its failure (frigidity).

Helene Deutsch (44, 45) has insisted upon the interval of time between the giving up of clitoris pleasure and the capacity for vaginal pleasure, which can develop only with puberty. However, the fantasy of being penetrated, of receiving, is present from the Oedipus phase. This interval, during which the vagina is not perceived as an erotic receptor, would explain, at least partly, the content of infantile fantasies about intercourse, pregnancy, and childbirth. Children spontaneously imagine that fertilization is an oral process, and that pregnancy is intestinal, the foetus being more or less assimilated to the faecal mass. 'Cloacal confusion' thus underlies fantasies of childbirth. Generally speaking, both intercourse and childbirth are visualized as bloody and painful since they are believed to involve bodily rupture. We shall see later how this explanation requires to be complemented.

Somewhat oversimplifying, we may say that, for the little girl, the Oedipus problem is a double one. She must change her love object (from mother to father) and her aim (from clitoris pleasure, with its masculine characteristics, to vaginal pleasure, which can only be anticipated). The feeling of having been castrated leads to the desire to be 'like the mother' and to receive the father's child. But this compensatory desire implies the acceptance of masochistic and passive tendencies, since the first identification with the mother is with a 'castrated' mother.

A few comments will suffice to indicate that the Oedipus problem as it is experienced is dependent upon earlier object-relations,

26

especially the mother-daughter relationship during the stages of development known as the oral, anal, and phallic stages (100).

In the first place, a number of writers such as Jones, Karen Horney, Helene Deutsch, and Melanie Klein, emphasize the early stage at which a sense – if not a clear idea – of the vagina appears. This 'sense' refers back to the fantasy representation of the vaginal function symbolized by the earliest sucking activity, and to the pleasure that it provides. On the other hand, there is the problem of why the little girl should experience such a degree of frustration when she discovers the difference between the sexes. The so-called culturalist interpretation maintains that the 'inferiority' of the clitoris and the associated frustration are related to the cultural value attributed to masculinity and its representative symbol, the possession of a penis.

But psychoanalytic thinking has also taken another direction: the little girl believes herself to have possessed a penis which she has lost. Castration is felt as a reprisal or punishment. Punishment from whom, and for what? Not for masturbation itself, but for the fantasies accompanying it, fantasies which, at the earliest stages of development, concern the mother, but the mother perceived as a *phallic figure*. We thus come back to the problem of the primitive relation with the mother, which Melanie Klein has helped us to understand (82). This relation is marked by the extreme ambivalence which is characteristic of the oral phase, with its oscillation between the merging satisfaction of repletion and destructive, cannibalistic aggressiveness. This aggressiveness is regarded sometimes as primary, sometimes as the result of inevitable frustrations. One can see to what abyss the little girl's frustration regarding her clitoris refers: it revives early patterns which she seems to recapitulate in some way. This is why, as Freud points out (45), the giving up of masturbation is abrupt and its repression intense: it might revive a certain type of extremely anxious relationship with the mother. At the Oedipus stage, the little girl turns away from her mother in a movement of rejection which is marked by the clearest hostility, because, underlying the castration anxiety, there emerge more primitive fears of body fragmentation, of destruction, of annihilation, in response to destructive fantasies projected onto the mother. But it may be observed that these are also the anxieties of the little boy; and this enables us to understand more fully the basis of psychoanalytic views on the famous 'penis envy': its intensity is such precisely because it is a reaction formation, i.e.

27

because it offers a defence against more primitive and deeply repressed desires.

We have discussed these aspects of the oral stage at some length
only because their reactivation is often particularly clear during
pregnancy and, of course, suckling. It can readily be understood that
the similarity between the two situations (a generation apart) is most
likely to revive the first identifications of the parturient woman with
her mother and the related problems of aggressiveness and guilt, in
similar dyads formed by 'the child she has and the mother she is – the
child she was and the mother she had' (Racamier, 134, pp. 528 and
543).

We have already referred to the connexion between baby and
faecal mass in the little girl's fantasies. This takes us back to the
problems of the anal stage when eroticism is centred upon the anal
orifice, associated first with expulsion and then with retention, with its
implications of active mastery. This provides the basic pattern for
anxiety-laden questions about what is inside the body and has to
come out. Such fears have to do both with the body threatened by
retention (poison) or by evacuation (laceration), and with the object
expelled, whether because it is 'lost' or destroyed (castration) or
because it may be harmful or destructive. These fantasies will also
be powerfully mobilized during pregnancy and confinement.

What has already been said is sufficient to draw attention to the
complex way in which woman's reproductive functions are organized.
Two additional factors in post-Oedipal development make them
particularly vulnerable: the time-lag and the cultural opposition with
which they have to contend (Racamier, 132, p. 1).

In early childhood and up to puberty, cultural patterns favour the
acceptance of femininity. It is of particular interest to know whether
the little girl has adopted the play appropriate to her sex (dolls, etc.)
and the roles and reactions expected of her (mother-substitute in the
case of the elder sister, feminine affectation, etc.). But failure to
integrate the feminine role is to be seen particularly when menstruation appears. As Langer has emphasized (93, 94), the first menstruation is of extreme importance. It should, as Racamier remarks (132,
p. 1), 'be experienced by the normal adolescent with feelings of
joy and enthusiasm since it is the first real evidence of the advent of
womanhood and fertility'. This seldom happens in our culture,

28

however. Even if cases for which the beginning of menstruation is genuinely traumatic are excluded, there is frequently a certain ambivalence. To accept menstruation is, for the girl, to accept the fact that she will become a mother like her own mother, to achieve emancipation, and to give up the passive satisfactions of early childhood. But the complex problems raised by the girl's identification with her mother in her sexual and reproductive roles are by no means wholly overcome at puberty. Menstruation is therefore often experienced in a regressive way: in so far as it involves a discharge of blood, it may be equated with urinary or faecal excretion, with the associated disgust or guilt. Above all, it may serve as a reminder of the injury of castration.

We shall not consider in detail Helene Deutsch's observations on pre-puberty and the stage of puberty (44, Vol. 1, pp. 1–153). The re-awakening of inner drives does mean a recasting of the whole structure of the personality, with all the regressive and integrative possibilities that this implies. The obvious problems connected with endocrine and autonomic disturbances have their counterpart in the body-image, which is significantly altered by the development of the breasts.

However important this maturing crisis may be, it is not the last, since the first experience of motherhood is still to come. Moreover, the matured functions cannot come into operation immediately, since a latency period of purely cultural and social origin is imposed upon the girl before marriage and maternity. It is well known that the cultural prohibitions during this period are more stringent for girls than for boys. Finally, with regard to the psychosexual development of woman, problematical and temporally widely extended as it is, one should remember the danger presented by defloration, as well as the basic fact that, in women, there is no necessary association between orgasm and reproduction, and that, in consequence, sexual pleasure is less directly connected with the biological function than in man, and thus more influenced by cultural choice and values.

The most important aspects of this brief account of the psycho-analytic point of view may be summarized as follows:

Conflict is normal: this implies a dynamic view of the process of development, through fruitful regressions and crises of integration.

Normal and pathological are therefore continuous and differ not in nature but in degree. This enables us to approach pregnancy and childbirth from a comprehensive point of view, in so far as the whole idea of a normal-pathological threshold is questioned. This view differs from that of Bibring, who regards the threshold as being simply raised.

PREGNANCY AND CONFINEMENT

Maternity has been described above as an integrative stage, the nature of which – as a crisis – implies the revival of past conflicts. *Whether these have been satisfactorily resolved or not*, they must inevitably, for every woman, colour the content of this stage and influence in advance its meaning and the particular difficulties which threaten its development. For every woman the specific constellation of her personality revives these elements, but unequally, according to her prevailing defence mechanisms. What we wish to stress is that, in this context, external clinical observation is insufficient. An uneventful pregnancy cannot automatically be assumed to indicate a successful integration, but, at most, a certain type of defence mechanism which might well have damaging effects at a different level. It does not follow that because pregnancy constitutes a crisis the best way to deal with it is to neutralize it, although this is one way of handling it. The concept of fruitful regression implies a subtle dialectical process the clinical approach to which must be both highly individual and highly dynamic. This development through conflict to which we have already referred constitutes the ground on which every woman elaborates the pattern of her motherhood. To talk to a primipara of the 'child-penis' or of the 'father's child' is not an explanation or an end, but a starting-point. Similarly, the account that follows may be regarded as representing, as it were, the least common denominator of the psychic processes and the possible meanings of pregnancy and childbirth. This common denominator, of course, finds concrete expression only at the level of the structure of each woman's personality.

PREGNANCY

The first stage

At a deep symbolic level, pregnancy is the prolongation of coitus, and thus retains some of its meaning, the incorporated object (the sperm) directly 'representing' the man's penis and the man himself (Ferenczi,

30

53). In short, physical incorporation is accompanied by psychic incorporation. The significance of this incorporation is varied and the reactions that it stimulates are various according to the acceptance or rejection of pregnancy, the marital relationship, and so on. At this stage, however, manifestations of an oral type are prevalent and this provides both a reminder and a justification of the little girl's archaic idea of pregnancy as the result of oral impregnation. Nausea, vomiting, food cravings, boulimia, and hypersalivation may all be considered as variations on the theme of oral ambivalence. Nausea can be interpreted as a somatic equivalent of disgust at being pregnant; vomiting as a displaced, oral attempt at abortion; and cravings as compulsive symptoms intended to relieve – through symbolic fertilization – the anxiety provoked by the unconscious desire to terminate pregnancy.

Experiences at the anal stage reveal themselves by a tendency to constipation, expressing the prevalence of normal tendencies to retention, the failure of which could account for attacks of diarrhoea or even miscarriages at this stage. Furthermore, the unconscious equation of the child with the intestinal contents may engender disgust which is displaced onto objects in the outside world (for example, phobias of small animals).

At this stage, however, when the foetus is quasi-continuous with the mother's body, one often finds feelings of triumphant plenitude which reminds one of the idea of the infant-penis coming to fill in the initial incompleteness. These manifestations have, in general, the same structure as neurotic symptoms, i.e. they express both unconscious desires and the defences erected against the anxiety which is provoked by the reactivation of such desires.

The appearance of the first movements

This is an important moment, since it permits and indeed requires, even more uncompromisingly, the transcending of the early quasi-constant ambivalence. The perception of the actual existence of the child is accompanied by the disappearance of the transitional symptoms and the establishment of a relatively stable equilibrium, one might almost say, a kind of cruising speed.

The overall change in the personality results from the narcissistic inflexion of the libido, i.e. the libido is withdrawn from either the external world as a whole or from particular areas. The woman turns in upon herself, loving and confusing her body and her foetus, whose anabolism demands all her energies. Some pregnancies are thus experienced as extremely gratifying in a thoroughly narcissistic fusional way. At the other extreme, some women whose narcissism is too centred upon an unimpaired and unalterable body have difficulty in accepting these changes and suffer with respect to their body-image.

We must also, however, give due consideration to the other aspect of the psychic structure of the pregnant woman. The actual existence of the baby implies the development of a primary object-relationship, an anticipation of the subsequent separation. Complex processes of identification to which we have already referred are brought into action. Identification with the child reactivates the archaic relationship of the woman with her own mother, and all the problems that this involves.

In its negative aspects (anxiety and symptoms) as in its positive aspects (wellbeing and protection), the experience of pregnancy is regressive. The general tone is primarily oral, as indicated by the existence of hypersomnia, interest in food, greed, dependence and susceptibility in relation to the environment. This regression may not be well tolerated if it revives former anxiety or feelings of guilt. It may be exaggerated, passive needs appearing insatiable. However the case may be, character problems may assume troublesome proportions. We shall not consider here the frankly pathological problems of hyperemesis or puerperal psychoses. The interested reader may consult Brisset and Held (21) on this subject.

The end of pregnancy

This is marked essentially by the reactivation of ambivalence concerning retention and expulsion. While the woman has difficulty in surrendering all claims to possess the object and in abandoning the narcissistic gratifications of this merging relationship, the object-relationship to the coming child and the desire to see him born acquire strength. Timely delivery requires a slight prevalence of expulsive forces over retentive trends. This ambivalence between expulsion and retention is linked with the re-cathexis of the outside world, as revealed in the often compulsive preparation of the layette and accommodation for the baby, which is reminiscent of the instinctive nesting behaviour of certain birds.

CONFINEMENT

If maternity as a whole is a crisis, confinement may be regarded as its peak. We shall see how forcibly, as such, it articulates the regressive and progressive potentialities of the crisis and thus represents a crucial engagement of opposing forces. Its character as an *event*, temporally limited and biologically defined, helps to isolate it either as an exhilarating achievement or as a moment to be excluded from the woman's experience.

The progressive value of childbirth, upon which painless childbirth lays so much emphasis, is also stressed in psychoanalytic literature. It is, according to Racamier, 'the greatest thing a woman can do, something from which she can draw an enriching feeling of personal achievement' (132, p, 2.). For psychoanalysis, as we have seen, maternity is a process that involves conflicts, and its success depends upon the resolution and integration of these conflicts. From this point of view, birth appears as the final result of a struggle and may be valued as a triumph over all the fears and anxieties connected with the regressive potentialities of childbirth. Confinement, in fact, marks the end of the narcissistic merging period of pregnancy, during which the woman feels that she and her baby are one. Bodily separation from the child, even though it prolongs and ensures the object-relationship already begun, cannot fail, at a certain level, to be experienced as trauma, rupture, or castration, with all its anxiety-producing content, the historical origins of which have already been referred to. At this level, these refer mainly to the anal stage. Delivery in particular must allow the free expression of deep-seated tendencies to rejection, of an aggressive, destructive nature. Failure to integrate these tendencies, and their excessive repression, may make efforts at expulsion impossible because of early experience of sphincter control. Anxieties are also revived concerning the actual passage, and these may have to do with threats either to the child or to the mother's body. Such anxieties prolong the anxieties of pregnancy, especially those that concern possible defects in the child, and are directly connected with the mother's ambivalence towards the coming baby.

Birth may also be experienced as a regression of the deepest kind, in so far as the parturient woman identifies with her child and relives the trauma of her own birth (Rank, 135). In fact, fantasies connected with birth always involve two experiences of birth: that of the child and

33

4

that of the mother herself (Deutsch and Freud, 45). Here again arises the problem of the maternal relationship and the anxieties that remain attached to it.

Finally, the most extreme psychoanalytic views on childbirth concern the equivalence of childbirth and ejaculation, thus extending the equation of pregnancy with coitus. Here we find raised in the most striking way the problem of the articulation of pleasure, anxiety, and pain. Deutsch writes that, for the woman, 'confinement would be an orgy of masochistic pleasure' (43). Racamier thinks that 'some exceptionally relaxed women experience intense orgasmic pleasure although most of them deny it' (132, p. 2). But orgasm would be closely associated with the release of destructive instincts. These, according to Freud (58), would reach their highest level when the sexual instincts are satisfied. This would be the case in childbirth and would explain the depth and frequency of the fear of death found among parturient women, more adequately than the simple recognition of the fact that childbirth is an obviously bloody process.

In touching upon the ultimate, metapsychological implications of psychoanalysis, we may appear to have left clinical reality a long way behind. It is useful, however, to draw attention to these implications since they give the problem of childbirth anxiety its setting, not in terms of simple cultural conditioning, but in terms of fundamental conflicts bound to the human psyche. Pain, for example, associated as it is with anxiety, is only one of the possible modes of response that the organism may use. We shall return to this point in Chapter 3.

From this point of view, if childbirth represents a decisive experience, or culminating point, this can only be in so far as it supports archaic anxieties. It holds promise in so far as it holds threat. Like pregnancy, it provides the occasion for fruitful regression.

Childbirth undeniably reduces the cohesion and strength of the ego, as indeed this regression indicates. The modes of adjustment and the defence mechanisms brought into action in response to this regressive situation are varied. The woman has to adjust to a biological process, to the behaviour required of her by the environment, and to the new situation created by the arrival of the child. Only the last of these can be schematically described, in terms of two coexisting emotional trends.

The negative trend involves a feeling of severe loss, a disappointment, sometimes a sense of paradise lost bound up with identification with the child.

The positive trend comprises, first, a brief phase dominated by a feeling of victorious achievement; and then, the relationship to the child, which cancels the negative trend and extends the relationship from its previous prenatal form with a speed proportional to the degree of accuracy with which it is anticipated. The relationship to the child does not always develop easily from the start, even in favourable cases, contrary to the opinion of Gressot (66, p. 72). It is better established with suckling, which re-establishes a relative merging with the mother. Adjustment to the existence of the child by sight and touch is sometimes accompanied by a certain stupor, a slight feeling of strangeness. This is, however, less marked than in the case of women delivered under anaesthesia.

According to the psychoanalytic point of view, therefore, childbirth at every level and at every stage proceeds on a groundwork of anxiety.

At the beginning of the present chapter we raised the question of the value of psychoanalytic theory in a study which, as we shall see later, is intended to provide statistical evidence on childbirth and its determinants.

The first conclusion to which our all too brief review leads us is that such research is justified. Obstetrically, childbirth is a limited and clearly defined biological phenomenon. The psychological perspective of preparation is based on this 'unity'. The psychoanalytic point of view, in emphasizing the manifold basic meanings of childbirth, is not opposed to such a delimitation. Consequently, the following hypotheses can be advanced:

Childbirth, in its various psychosomatic aspects, and through deeplying tendencies, represents an extension of the woman's personal development and, in particular, of her earliest object-relationships and the stages of her instinctual maturation.

Confinement may be of some importance for studying the structure of the mother-child relationship, the subsequent effects of which are, at the present time, generally emphasized. The question still remains, of course, whether it is the confinement as such that affects the quality of this relationship, or whether the confinement *and* the

35

relationship are connected only because of common determining factors.

Wherever the truth may lie, it seems reasonable to accept that confinement may have diagnostic and prognostic value in so far as it may reveal deep-lying determining factors which may also affect the subsequent mother-child relationship. But confinement is influenced by other factors at very different levels (for example, preparation or obstetrical factors), and may, by its very quality as act and experience, *redirect* the trend of the woman's life and *reorient* her outlook.

These two attitudes must always be kept clearly in mind. On the one hand, childbirth must be seen in relation to the more or less closed network of determining factors which give it meaningful continuity with both past and future. On the other hand, one must bear in mind the possibility of appreciating the dynamic potential that belongs to childbirth just by reason of its relative contingency.

These considerations give rise directly to the methodological problems of what childbirth is, what its supposed determinants are, and how these can be handled in statistically based research. The following chapters will demonstrate the extreme complexity of these problems. For the moment, it may be helpful to make one or two observations:

(a) As far as investigation is concerned, it must be emphasized that the 'critical' nature of pregnancy and childbirth enables relatively deep material to be collected more readily than in other circumstances. This, of course, in no way prejudices validity.

(b) For a conceptual approach to the problems involved, a number of ideas directly inspired by psychoanalysis are useful and indeed indispensable: for example, intrapsychic conflict, ambivalence, unconscious guilt, introjected imagos (especially maternal), body-image, and ego defence mechanisms.

(c) Consequently, in the face of these extremely difficult problems, three main lines of investigation seem to offer some possibility of enlarging the scope of the data usually collected.

Thus:

(i) The concept of a physiological or 'ballistic' approach to childbirth is related to, and placed in the context of, a psychosomatic framework which includes the ideas of anxiety and body-image.

(ii) The concept of the relationship with the staff of the labour ward (the objective importance of which is often exaggerated) requires reference to be made to psychological data relating to the prior cathexis by the woman of the experience to come, according to her predominant defence mechanisms.

(iii) The pseudo-objective concept of pain extends to that of suffering and consequently to those of anxiety and of pleasure (moral or erogenous masochism).

Before concluding this chapter, we must refer to the sociocultural aspect, although it does not concern us directly. In fact, the concept of crisis allows us conveniently to summarize this problem. Precisely in so far as we speak of the crisis of maternity we are referring to a problem which is neither specific to a particular woman nor entirely a function of her personal past experience, but is a universal and there-fore anthropological problem. Discussions about the painful or pain-less nature of childbirth among primitive peoples have at least had the merit of showing that, beyond this limited aspect of pain and the considerable variations to be found in this respect, childbirth and maternity are universally ritualized (Mead and Newton, 106). Neither birth nor death has ever, anywhere, been regarded entirely as a 'natural' phenomenon. On the contrary, birth provides an ideal opportunity for understanding the way in which culture enmeshes the crucial facts of nature in a symbolic network (Mead, 105).

It is, of course, always possible to 'show' that the response elabor-ated by each culture only shifts the question while keeping it open. The attribution of cultural significance blocks but also awakens anxiety, conceals but also expresses the human situation. It can readily be shown, as we hope to prove in Chapter 3, that painless childbirth serves a similar purpose in present-day society.

SUMMARY

Chapter 2 summarizes psychoanalytic theories of motherhood, pregnancy, and childbirth in their topical and dynamic aspects. Such theories can be understood only if the major stages in woman's psychosexual development are borne in mind. Maternity appears as an integrative crisis. If it is to enable the maternal role to be assumed in the actual mother-child relationship, it must also involve the revival of the structuring conflicts which have marked the mother's personal history and moulded her identifications.

Childbirth is the 'end' – at least a temporary one – of this crisis, and also frequently its culminating point. The way in which it is experienced depends upon the woman's whole past history; at the same time, it is exposed to the hazards of a crucial moment in time, and may have a directive effect on the future. Childbirth, charged thus with the many conscious and unconscious meanings with which psychoanalysis endows it, may be regarded as a proper and particularly interesting subject for research from this point of view, as well as from that of obstetrics and preparation.

CHAPTER 3

Problems in the Study of Childbirth

The previous chapter has shown us that, from the point of view of depth psychology, childbirth – even though its characteristics may be less circumscribed and limited than would appear in obstetrics – can defensibly be identified, as a field of research, at two levels:

At the diagnostic level, in as much as the confinement is not independent of the course of the woman's life-history, it is a process governed by complex psychosomatic interactions, which it may indeed bring to light.

At the prognostic level, the course of the confinement and the way in which it is experienced and acted have undoubted importance for the mother's psychic economy and the future mother-child relationship. Our research is not directed towards this aspect, although this assumption is implicitly recognized.[1]

The research is centred upon the study of the determining factors of childbirth conceived as a psychosomatic process, and upon the manner in which the integration of such factors with preparation for childbirth will modify the course of events.

Such a study immediately encounters two kinds of problem with which we shall deal successively in the present chapter.

The first concerns the assessment of childbirth itself. If confinements are to be compared and related to previous personal factors, we must define the headings and concepts used to evaluate confinements and the childbirth patterns that may eventually emerge. A review of the literature on childbirth viewed as an isolated sector will serve to illustrate the difficulties raised by the definition and quantification of the necessary variables. This review will also serve as a justification of the provisional solution of these difficulties that we have adopted (cf. section on childbirth, pp. 40–54).

[1] Appendix II, Section III, p. 273.

The second problem is that of objectifying past personal factors which may eventually be found to be determinant. This is a problem of a more general nature: the classification of material obtained prior to confinement must be relevant to the classification used for the confinement itself, while it is, of course, also dependent upon the empirical method of investigation adopted. It was obvious, from the start, that these determinants were many and varied. One may wonder, for example, what there is in common between global classifications of character and a methodical inventory of the psychosomatic semiology of pregnancy. Yet both can be related to the process of childbirth. This gives an idea of the innumerable possible lines of investigation, each of which requires a specific approach. Previous work done on this problem, which is reviewed in Appendix II, illustrates the extreme diversity of the methodologies adopted. We shall be concerned here, however, only with those that can be adapted to the conditions of our own research, on the one hand, and that are relevant to childbirth, on the other. In the present chapter, therefore, we shall refer only to research studies that have included childbirth among their principal concerns (cf. section on factors in childbirth, pp. 54–68).

We shall also make use of several studies on maternity, the methodological interest of which is patent. It must be emphasized that we draw on these works only to illustrate the methodological difficulties, irrespective of the interest of their hypotheses and the results obtained. The reader interested in the content of these studies may refer to the review in Appendix II.

CHILDBIRTH

The first difficulty is to decide how childbirth can be *evaluated*.

In the previous chapter we saw that childbirth represented a psychological event of particular significance, a critical period associated with the well-defined nature of the biological event. We reminded the reader of the deep unconscious meaning of delivery itself. But more immediately, from the standpoint of present-day psychology, how is it viewed? Most frequently, childbirth is seen as a possible trauma. We shall not elaborate this point of view, or seek to discover whether it corresponds to the serious biological threat that delivery has entailed and still entails, or whether it is a cultural

40

phenomenon. It will be sufficient to emphasize that, with the idea of trauma as the starting-point, childbirth must necessarily be apprehended through two complementary indices which embody its problems in a realistic and positive manner, pain and behaviour.

Pain

Pain cannot, today, be conceived as the result of an objective percept. Rof-Carballo, for example (quoted by Ajuriaguerra, 3), defines pain as follows: 'Pain is a *reaction* as well as a perception, and at the same time a form of *expression*, highly individualized and varying from person to person, and an emotional *manifestation* dependent upon the subject's personal experience and past history. The accompanying centrifugal reactions are substantially related to pain.'

In spite, however, of the many contributions of surgeons, neurologists, and psychologists, underlining the complexity and the subjective nature of this phenomenon, there remains a tendency to use the word 'pain' in the sense of a response to an external or internal stimulus, which is objective and measurable. This usage of the term corresponds to a certain need for positive thinking; it also makes it possible to distinguish 'pain', as a simple isolated factor, from 'suffering', which refers to the whole being and expresses a mode of experience.

But once this definition is accepted, the 'objective' phenomenon of pain tends to conceal accompanying problems. This is made particularly clear in the approach to childbirth where pain seems to crystallize all impending threats. It becomes the focus for projections of the deep-seated anxiety it releases. Pain simply seems to be the incarnation of everything 'bad' about childbirth, which thus becomes an event somehow exterior to the parturient woman. It is a sort of 'trial', the difficulty of which is directly proportional to the amount of pain connected with the biological process of delivery.

Behaviour

We now come to our second index, behaviour. In the first instance, behaviour is the resultant of two factors: on the one hand, the intensity of the pain, which should, ideally, be measurable; on the other hand, the woman's inner resources, especially qualities of moral character such as courage, stoicism, and a readiness for self-sacrifice for the benefit of the newborn, or psychophysiological qualities such as strength, stamina, and endurance. It is in this context that extreme and abnormal forms of behaviour have, in the past, been described (the classic wrath of parturient women, for example).

As soon as the illusion of an objective measure of pain is destroyed, it can be seen how arbitrary this concept is. Moreover, extreme forms of behaviour cannot be regarded simply as the outward expression of a painful 'percept'. In fact, they raise the problem of a comprehensive approach to psychopathology, which would attempt to apprehend the specific nature of each parturient woman's experience, in the light of her past history. This kind of understanding might be envisaged for all parturient women, even for those who show no exaggerated forms of behaviour.

In short, if we stop regarding pain as the result of a measurable stimulus, we are inevitably led to view it as a reaction, or form of expression, or emotion. This means that it can be apprehended only in terms of a meaningful structure which is more or less specific to each woman. Thus we come up against the general problem of the limitations of behaviourism. It is, however, scarcely possible to evaluate confinements and compare them with one another without continuing to use the concepts of pain and behaviour, though we can, at least, bear in mind their relativity and their limitations.

In the next section, we shall examine the standpoint of obstetricians and practitioners of the PPM, with a view to selecting those elements that may be of use in our research.

CHILDBIRTH FROM THE STRICTLY OBSTETRICAL POINT OF VIEW

Theoretically, the orthodox obstetrician is little interested in the psychological aspects of childbirth. We do not mean to imply that in his actual practice he overlooks any of the woman's reactions or fails to learn from experience how to manage them. But this knowledge is not directed towards any systematic or theoretical approach. It is, in fact, part of the 'art' of establishing good relationships, which is every practitioner's aim.

This being so, we must inquire how this strictly obstetrical position can be defined. In summary, it may be said that childbirth, like pregnancy, although not an illness, does imply possible dangers and risks for the mother and especially for the child. The ideal is therefore childbirth *without* complications and, from this point of view, confinement is defined in negative terms. What becomes, then, of pain and behaviour? What the obstetrician expects is that the mother's behaviour will not disturb the physiological process, and the control he has over it. If he tries to suppress pain he does so, it is true, as a humanitarian obligation, but more precisely, technically speaking, it is because pain may cause harmful behaviour and may also affect uterine activity. Suppression of pain is, however, a secondary aim and remains strictly subordinate to considerations of safety. The main ambition of 'scientific' obstetrics is the entirely directed confinement in which the process is under the complete control of the responsible obstetrician.

It may be noted incidentally that such a position is not without advantages: deep-seated anxieties released during childbirth could be reduced to a rational apprehension of the biological threat, which, in turn, has been greatly attenuated by the appreciable progress of obstetrics, as represented by the obstetrician. Thus, theoretically, childbirth could be entirely neutralized, and deprived of all emotional significance and tension. This would appear to be one of the trends in scientific obstetrics, especially in America. Its implications and consequences remain to be seen.

If this 'strictly' obstetrical point of view is accepted, the objective criteria for the evaluation of childbirth remain to be ascertained. At a macroscopic level, a good confinement, in this perspective, would be defined by the absence of 'complications', either for the mother (tearing, haemorrhage, etc.) or for the child (foetal injury indicated by abnormal heart beat, and later by the actual condition of the newborn child: colour, appearance, crying, meconium, or need for resuscitation).

These criteria are of unquestionable objective value. But as soon as a more differentiated mode of evaluation is required, methodological difficulties of two kinds arise. On the one hand, certain recordable facts (for example, an episiotomy) can differ in their obstetrical significance; on the other, and above all, they may be as much a reflection of the attitude adopted by the obstetrician (towards the indication for an episiotomy, for example) as of the physiological process itself. In other words, indications for such interventions as forceps, episiotomy, or medication are not sufficiently precise to constitute a basis for a truly objective differentiation of confinements. Obstetrical 'management' is, finally, a function not only of the

43

obstetrical problems relevant to each woman, but also of the obstetrician's technique and the specific circumstances surrounding each confinement, which do not lend themselves to systematic classification (midwives' reports, number of women in the labour ward and its prevailing atmosphere, etc.)

The purpose of these remarks is only to emphasize the difficulty of establishing a set of discriminative and valid variables for the evaluation of childbirth from a strictly obstetrical point of view. Such a set of variables would have to take normal confinement as its point of reference; and normal confinement may be defined as taking place within flexible but comparable limits of time, its progression being uniform. Evaluation would take into account the total length of time involved, which should be neither too long nor too short, the duration of each stage (dilatation, transition, expulsion, issue), the regularity of progression, and the quality and intensity of the rhythmic uterine contractions. A detailed report of the newborn infant's condition – especially anoxia – would also be of major importance.

One can appreciate the complexity of the problems involved in assembling all this material, rating it according to a pre-established reference scale, and eventually combining the various aspects to provide a general assessment of childbirth in obstetrical terms.

After several attempts and lengthy reflection, it became clear to us that a really elaborate classification of confinements along these lines was impossible. We therefore adopted a simple form of scoring which enabled us to distinguish three groups of confinements:

> One group consists of cases with such serious obstetrical complications that it is impossible, from the start, to compare them with others in respect of pain, behaviour, or determinants of a psychosomatic kind. Frank organic dystocias may be taken as examples of this group.

> At the other extreme is a group consisting of 'normal' confinements. This group does, of course, include a wide range of obstetrical data, but these data do not contribute to explaining the other parameters of childbirth (pain, behaviour).

> The third group is an intermediate one: it contains all the confinements in which 'incidents' occurred, but the psychological implications of these incidents cannot be ruled out *a priori* (cervical

dystocias, borderline indication for forceps, blood transfusion, etc.).

PSYCHOPROPHYLACTIC EVALUATION OF CHILDBIRTH

In Chapter 1, attention was drawn to ideas and facts concerning preparation for childbirth. We must now return to these, in so far as preparation is relevant to the present problem of how childbirth can be objectively evaluated. The effects of preparation may be considered at two levels:

(a) Factors that were already present in the obstetrical point of view (pain and behaviour), but were of only secondary importance, become of primary concern and must thereby lend themselves to quantification.

(b) The aims of preparation for childbirth have introduced, more or less explicitly, a number of psychological concepts which have, up to a point, modified the whole approach to the evaluation of childbirth.

Pain and behaviour

In a sense, preparation may be regarded simply as an extension of obstetrical research on effective and danger-free methods of analgesia; and we have already seen why pain and behaviour provide the most tangible factors for a psychological evaluation of childbirth. Thus preparation, in so far as it had to demonstrate its effectiveness, emphasized these factors and the need to quantify them.

The first research workers used a five-point scale, for pain only, ranging from complete analgesia to complete failure. In the absence of a perfect instrument for measuring pain, values on the scale were assigned according to a rather heterogeneous selection of indices, including the parturient woman's moaning, her behaviour in so far as it seemed to 'express' pain, and her own appraisal after delivery.

Later, confronted with frequent differences between sometimes impeccable behaviour and allegations or limited expressions of severe pain, certain authors divided the scale into two parts, one for assessing pain, the other for evaluating behaviour. Henceforth, the percentage of successes was on a much higher level according to the behavioural index than according to the pain index (28, p. 190).

45

Attempts were then made to improve the criteria for assessing analgesia. Jordania (79), for example, proposed three levels of intensity of pain:

severe pain, indicated by one or more of the following signs:
frequent crying out during contractions
agitation
grinding of the teeth
tears;

moderate pain, indicated by one or more of the following signs:
moaning
weak and intermittent cries
a look of discomfort;

mild pain, indicated by faint and infrequent moans (signs of severe and moderate pain being absent).

In addition, severe pain was considered to be present when one of the signs of moderate pain was associated with at least two of the following symptoms:

pupillary dilatation during contractions
acceleration of pulse and respiration
oliguria
hyperaemia of the skin and abdomen
rise in blood pressure of more than 10 mm Hg.

Critical observations. Anyone who has ever attempted to devise a scale for measuring pain and behaviour during childbirth is aware of the extreme difficulty of the task. Yet the need for such a scale is imperative. We can scarcely regard as satisfactory the manner in which the results of preparation are presented, and before we proceed to explain how we have used the double scale, a few remarks seem called for.

In the first place, there is the question whether retrospective impressions of the parturient woman, relative to pain, should be used. At first sight it might appear that nothing could be more useful, since what matters is, after all, the memory the mother retains of her confinement. Why, then, should we not make exclusive use of these descriptions, and compare them with one another?

Two objections can be made to this procedure, if we are to maintain our requirement for an objective, though approximate, evaluation of pain.

First, the processes integrating personal experience, deeply unconscious processes (repression, denial, aesthetic dramatization, etc.), are too varied and too personal for the painful event to retain even the appearance of an objective percept. This does not mean that the retrospective account of the confinement is of no interest for the assessment of pain; but, as we shall see later, its use would mean giving up the aim of objectivity.

Second, and more immediately, the very act of giving a retrospective account activates conscious motivations (thankfulness, gratitude, resentment) or unconscious motivations (return gift, exhibitionism, sense of modesty). These motivations deserve attention: they have not yet been studied but their existence provides a further reason for regarding a retrospective personal account of the 'painful sensations' of delivery as anything but objective.

Let us now turn to the objective observation of behaviour during childbirth. Here, we have to contend with two difficulties.

On the one hand, we might try to register every possible expression of pain. Such an *objective pain index* may be widely extended (ranging from cries to groans, from groans to wails, from wails to tears and grimaces). But it is well known that impassivity can be the most expressive evidence of pain. Moreover, the most refined set of materials for a pain index soon requires interpretation. The idea of pure objectivity must therefore be abandoned. The same could be said of autonomic manifestations such as pupillary dilatation: in view of the extreme diversity of the functions of the autonomic nervous system, these cannot be regarded as providing more 'objective' evidence of the presence of pain.

It should now be apparent that the attempt to construct a refined scale of pain by means of objective observations of behaviour rapidly leads to an impasse, owing to the absence of a valid scale of behaviour.

The other alternative, the assessment of behaviour with reference to *pre-established norms*, has its own disadvantages. These norms, in the perspective of preparation for childbirth, represent perfect models of behaviour envisaged by such preparation. They include, ideally, both the control of all negative manifestations (related to pain, anxiety, or any other affect) and the quality of the techniques acquired (breathing, relaxation, expulsion). But such norms can be applied only to expectant mothers who have been trained for preparation, and this constitutes a serious methodological disadvantage. In addition, these norms lack sufficient precision since they fail to discriminate between a kind of 'neutrality' of behaviour (which does not hinder the obstetrician) and a form of active adjustment (which may actually help him).

Our point of view. These observations will help the reader to understand the method we decided to adopt to solve this delicate problem of measuring pain and behaviour: we chose a double-scoring system, which takes into account the inevitable intrusion of subjective factors into objective evaluation.

The index of behaviour is as objective as possible and simply registers – by reference to an ideal norm of silence and relaxation – all *expressions of discomfort*, whether they result from pain or anxiety, from fear or exhibitionism, from organic injury or destructuring of the ego. It is, in other words, blind scaling, independent of any interpretation.

The pain index makes no claim to represent an objective evaluation of a simple phenomenon: it is deliberately interpretative and aims at reflecting the personal experience of 'suffering' as a whole. Scale values are based not only on direct observation and obstetrical data, but also on interviews, retrospective accounts, and clinical intuition of the modes of expression particular to each parturient woman.

In addition, there is a separate scale for the application of the techniques acquired during preparation.

It should not be forgotten that the results of preparation have been evaluated in obstetrical terms proper: reduction of the duration of labour, of complications (haemorrhage, shock, resuscitation), and of intervention (forceps, episiotomy, medication). The difficulties involved in the objective assessment of these factors have already been indicated: they derive from the involvement of the obstetrician's personal approach and from the flexibility of the criteria leading to various obstetrical indications.

Psychological values promulgated by the PPM

We have discussed above the problems raised by the need to quantify pain and behaviour if an objective assessment of confinement is to be made. But, as we have already stated, the aims of preparation for childbirth have also introduced psychological values, which widen our frame of reference. We propose to define these values before considering whether they can be incorporated into a scale for childbirth. These values are not always explicit in studies on psychoprophylaxis, but the main features are as follows.

Analgesia is not a sufficient end in itself. According to the theory of preparation, it is the concrete aspect or necessary condition of success. Success, however, may be defined differently, as the realization of a *conscious, happy,* even ecstatic confinement. These terms should be noted, since, ideally, it is they that should be quantified. Painless childbirth leads to new standards for childbirth: a good confinement implies *activity*, directed by means of a *technique*, resulting in behavioural *control* more or less *pain free* and allowing cooperation with the obstetrician; an emotional *participation* in the birth; and a *positive emotional relation* to the child, in the *joy* of *achievement*.

From the psychoprophylactic point of view, childbirth is not only a potentially negative moment: the wellbeing of the parturient woman does not consist solely in the *absence* of suffering or tearing, or in *not* having a *traumatized* child. Childbirth is an aim in itself, to be experienced as a positive moment in the woman's life, the main value of which consists in the activity that she puts into it.

In the light of the psychoanalytic views summarized in Chapter 2, we may make a few brief comments underlining the assumptions and limitations of this approach.

The *first assumption* is that the mere suppression of the negative affect involved in pain is sufficient to allow positive affect to develop. It is well known that this is the case only to a limited extent and that the problems of childbirth are highly complex. This is, however, of little practical importance. What must be stressed is the risk that may be involved in emphasizing these positive affects. If parturient women are required not only to show well-adjusted behaviour, but also to express joy and happiness, such demands may nourish feelings of guilt.

The *second assumption* is that, in the good confinement as defined from the standpoint of preparation, great importance is attached to the parturient woman's activity. Certain authors have pointed out the risk of promoting a form of 'masculine protest' with such a request for activity (cf. p. 9). Without going as far as this, the psychological limits of this notion of activity should be emphasized: every form of

49

activity is not necessarily 'good'. We have come across active and well-adjusted women whose activity led only to a kind of formal control, not only of behaviour, but of all genuine affect. In practice, it is not easy for midwives to handle confinements in the labour ward in the most usual manner, i.e. in a firm and directive manner, emphasizing the parturient woman's control, and, at the same time, to contemplate the possibility of introducing a more flexible, permissive, and tolerant attitude which might be of greater benefit in certain cases. The positive value of regressive and passive experiences, when they are well tolerated and accepted by other people, is well known. They represent one modality of 'corrective emotional experience'. *Every form of regression is not negative in itself.* Ideally these regressions 'in the service of the ego' should be respected, and even encouraged, in view of their *maturing value.* Finally, from a purely psychological point of view, childbirth may be evaluated through the concept of a *maturing experience,* in which regression and progression articulate in a strictly personal manner. Bibring *et al.* (14, 15) have emphasized the difficulty of judging the maturing value of an experience. Such a judgement implies an appreciation of the whole course of the woman's life, followed up after confinement; only a procedure such as this can apprehend the 'sense' of the confinement, at the deepest level. But such a personalized approach would make comparisons extremely difficult. What has just been said suggests that, in the last resort, preparation involves the risk of exacting strictly 'normal' behaviour, disregarding the potentially fruitful regressive tendencies of certain parturient women. Such attitudes, tinged with rigidity, refer to a kind of preparation that used to be strictly applied. Today, however, this kind of preparation is being abandoned for a more tolerant and flexible approach to childbirth (cf. Appendix II, Section IV, p. 275).

Research such as we have undertaken may therefore help practitioners of psychoprophylaxis to understand their patients better and to adapt preparation to their individual needs, partly by providing models for more elaborate and detailed anamnesis with regard to especially significant areas, partly by affording a better grasp of determining factors in childbirth and of the relations between the woman's previous history, her pregnancy, and her confinement.

The complexity of the problems raised by the introduction of psychological values into the appreciation of childbirth should now be clear. From a practical point of view, however, activity, relationship with the environment, and the immediate relationship with the child, must be recognized as important and significant factors for *any* objective evaluation of childbirth, and relevant data should be collected systematically. An account of the procedure adopted in the present research will be given later.

THE MAIN RESEARCH STUDIES ON CHILDBIRTH

The factors relevant for the assessment of childbirth from both obstetrical and psychoprophylactic points of view have already been indicated. A brief account will now be given of some investigations which have had to face this problem of assessment (whether of prepared or of unprepared childbirth). Our concern is confined to *the manner in which this problem has been dealt with* in these studies and disregards their hypotheses and results, although these no doubt constitute their main interest. As far as the precise problem of evaluation is concerned, we shall encounter again the ideas that we have already outlined.

Studies that make use of obstetrical data only

Ferreira (54) uses, for purposes of correlation, *duration of labour, type of anaesthesia*, and *type of delivery*. Rosengren (141, 142) refers to *duration* and to *difficulty* of delivery. Scott and Thompson (144) use *length, termination*, and *type of delivery*.

Studies that make use of both obstetrical and psychological data

Pleshette *et al.* (129) describe the women's *reactions* during labour. Davids *et al.* (41, 42) distinguish between women *who have difficulties* in the labour ward and those *who do not*. From an organic point of view they refer to the existence or absence of *defects* or *somatic complications in the infant*.

Winokur and Werboff (156) are interested in *psychological reactions* during childbirth and, in particular, use the concept of *tolerance*. Women were classified by the obstetrician according to three degrees of tolerance: the woman was considered to be tolerant if she showed few or no signs of fear, was anxious to end her labour, rarely asked for relief, seldom cried out, and showed cooperation in her efforts at bearing down; she was low in tolerance if she showed the opposite characteristics. In this research, another interesting obstetrical index was *the delay between the estimated and the actual date* of the confinement.

Newton (114, 115) uses two kinds of information: (a) obstetrical –
dose of anaesthetics and *percentage of analgesics*; (b) psychological –
emotional tone of the subsequent account given by the woman. Some
show negative feelings towards their confinement, others show
positive feelings.

Klein, Potter, and Dyk (83) classify childbirth in terms of: (a) *good*
or *bad* confinement (obstetrically speaking); (b) *positive* or *negative*
psychological *reaction*. For these authors, there is no direct relation
between the quality of the labour and that of the psychological
reaction; even anxiety-free women retain traumatic memories of their
confinement.

Pavenstedt, in research of major importance (123, 124), records and
classifies data as follows: (a) obstetrical – the obstetrician makes
detailed observations of labour, estimating its *intensity*, the difficulty
of *dilatation*, the effectiveness of *medication*, the *depth of anaesthesia*,
and possible sources of *foetal trauma*; (b) psychological – a member
of the research team is present until the woman has fully recovered
from the anaesthetic (which is an indication that anaesthesia is
systematically used) and records her *attitudes* and her *reactions* to
pain, medication, and *anaesthesia*. Particular attention is given to the
first *reaction of the mother towards her child.* A specialized observer
examines the baby.

A psychoanalytical approach

Finally, we may refer to the work of Malcovati *et al.* (101) who approach childbirth from a psychoanalytic point of view. They distinguish two forms of anxiety: paranoid anxiety connected with the
sense of personal danger, and depressive anxiety connected with the
sense of danger to the object. From the women's verbalization of
their confinements these authors establish an association between
depressive anxiety and dilatation, and between paranoid anxiety and
expulsion.

Such an attempt to distinguish the conflicts characteristic of each
phase of the confinement calls for the use of an analytical instrument
geared to the chronological course of the confinement. This, in fact, is
what we have done, as will presently be seen. It must be noted that
Malcovati *et al.*, although they distinguish between two *types* of

anxiety, give no indication as to the possibility of a *quantitative* assessment of anxiety.

It is evident that the various factors used for the evaluation of child-birth in the several works mentioned above are similar to those we had ourselves isolated and are subject to the same reservations, indicated below:

> *Obstetrical data* can readily be objectified only in elementary form. Furthermore, their discriminative value weakens as obstetrical indications become more systematic (for example, the use of medication, anaesthesia, and forceps, beyond a certain frequency, makes a classification of confinements impossible).

> *Psychological data* are of three kinds: behaviour as an expression of tolerance and control; the emotional tone of the subsequent ac-count; and psychological reactions. Each of these three types is extremely heterogeneous (see, for example, Winokur and Werboff's definition of tolerance, cited on p. 51).

An important observation has been made by Pleshette *et al.* (129). After having demonstrated that there is no relationship between prenatal anxiety and reactions during labour, these authors add that *this finding is invalid because reactions were weakened by the systematic administration of sedatives.* This would appear to be a fundamental point: a very directive and active management of confinements *prevents the appearance of psychological differences,* whether they concern behaviour, relationship to others, or relationship to the child. The characteristic of orthodox obstetrics, as we have seen, is a ten-dency to standardize childbirth procedures in the interests of better control. The same tendency appears at a different level in preparation for childbirth, in the form of a highly normative definition of appro-priate behaviour. This is a methodological problem of a general nature: a confinement can be evaluated, whether in obstetrical or in psychological terms, only within a certain frame of reference provided by the 'obstetrical style' of the obstetrician, including both his technique and what he 'expects' of the parturient woman.

To conclude this section, let us briefly summarize the factors that have been used, from different points of view, for the evaluation of childbirth:

    (i) various obstetrical factors

    (ii) behaviour during confinement (mastery and control of the traumatic experience)

    (iii) pain and experience of pain

    (iv) nature of relationship to others

    (v) nature of relationship to the child

    (vi) subsequent personal account, psychological reaction

    (vii) maturing experience.

These are very heterogeneous factors, each referring to a specific perspective and requiring a specific mode of evaluation. A detailed account will be given in Chapter 5 of the manner in which our own scaling system was established.

Finally, we should like to make two further important points. First, although all these factors may be used in classifying confinements, they refer to a great variety of possible determinants of childbirth. For example, behaviour during confinement and the style of relation to others are connected with the parturient woman's capacity for adjustment and indeed with her defence mechanisms and her prevailing object-relations. On the other hand, obstetrical factors and intensity of pain would refer to a different level: that of anxiety, of distortions of body-image, etc., i.e. to a strictly psychosomatic level. Thus the choice of any particular factor for assessing confinement will depend upon *prior hypotheses* concerning its determinants. It will also depend upon the existing possibilities for research, which limit the extent to which such pre-existing determining factors can be isolated.

Second, despite the influence of these pre-existing determinants in the choice of the factors for assessing confinement, it seems possible and desirable to carry out an internal analysis of confinement, using every available factor. Such an analysis might facilitate the establishment of relationships between, for example, obstetrical, behavioural, and interpersonal factors, at different stages of the confinement. Thus contingent patterns of childbirth might appear, on the basis of which subsequent research on psychosomatic determinants could proceed.

RESEARCH ON THE 'FACTORS' INVOLVED IN CHILDBIRTH

As we stated at the beginning of this chapter, it is not our intention to provide a comprehensive review of research on pregnancy and maternity, or to examine in detail the methodological problem set by the choice of variables, or rather the conditions for such a choice, which would make possible the relation of childbirth to antecedent personal factors. Our intention is simply to give a critical account of our own tools of investigation.

These tools necessarily depend upon the specific way in which data are collected, and this, in turn, depends upon the practical possibilities of the research. Between the clinical depth approach of psychoanalytic inspiration, and questionnaires, it is apparent that a wide range of positions exists, within which our research had to be oriented. Actually this range is far narrower than it first appears. While our ultimate aim is directed to the deep-lying psychological features which alone give the problems of motherhood their full significance, we were in fact obliged to limit both the number and the nature of our investigations, and to obtain material which lent itself to standardization and statistical treatment. We shall first examine studies directly focused on childbirth and then proceed to consider those which, being concerned with pregnancy and maternity, are thus indirectly relevant.

INVESTIGATIONS CENTRED UPON CONFINEMENT

Here we shall deal first with investigations carried out within the framework of preparation, and then with those conducted outside this frame of reference.

Within the frame of reference of preparation

By adopting the concept of nervous type, the Russian authors have attempted to bring a degree of precision to the prognosis of success in the psychoprophylactic method.

Nicolaiev (117, 118) and his school attempt to elaborate a method for determining the nervous type of expectant mothers, on the basis of the Pavlovian fourfold classification: strong unbalanced type, strong balanced type, strong balanced slow type, and weak unbalanced type. In addition to the strength, quality, and nature of the relations between excitation and inhibition, these authors also try to take into consideration certain peculiarities of the relations between the first and second signalling systems and between the cortex and the sub-cortical area.

55

To begin with, the method elaborated by Astakhov and Beskrovnaia (6) was based upon:

detailed anamnesis

observation of behaviour during both preparation and confinement

a study of suggestibility

a study of the relationship between inhibition and excitation in the word association test (Gakkel)

a plethysmographic record.

The anamnesis consisted of a detailed investigation of the following points:

the social background in which the expectant mother was brought up

her relationships with her parents, friends, and relatives

her school record

her professional activity, how she started off, her liking for work

her capacity for adjusting to new tasks or a new environment

her relations with her husband, his parents, and his friends

her attitude towards children in general, towards her own children in particular, and towards her pregnancy.

Special attention was given to the following:

capacity for work

perseverance

initiative

ability to learn

interest in social matters

capacity for concentration

adjustment to new tasks

self-control

attitudes to danger

ingenuity

adjustment to a new environment

capacity for communication

sensitiveness

preoccupation with health

manner of presenting her symptoms

cleanliness, tidiness

calmness

attentiveness

irritability
capacity for distraction
anxiety, impatience, agitation
importunity
speed of falling asleep and awakening.

In view of the subjective nature of these data, additional sources of information (parents, friends, etc.) were used with the help of a social worker.

Behaviour during preparation and confinement was recorded 'in collaboration with the staff of the maternity ward'. Suggestibility was assessed by the eyelid test and Nicolaiev's test, which is similar to the body-sway test.

Jordania (79) presented at the Congress of Kiev (37) another method for determining the typological characteristics of expectant mothers (see *Table 4*).

Levit and Rabinovitch (97) have also attempted to study nervous type on the basis of anamnestic data and observation of the expectant mother's behaviour. They point out that their method is incomplete because of the 'subjective character of the information obtained by questioning'. These results give information on the 'emotional make-up' of the expectant mother rather than on her typological character-istics.

The use of this method in the prognosis of confinement has given the following results:

Result	Predicted cases	Observed cases
Excellent	656 (51·8%)	546 (43·2%)
Good	424 (33·4%)	412 (32·6%)
Indifferent	164 (12·9%)	197 (19·6%)
No effect	22 (1·9%)	35 (2·7%)

There appears to be a strong prevalence of the weak unbalanced type among the poor results.

Critical comments. We shall not dwell upon the inadequacy of Pavlov's nervous types as applied to human clinical problems. This

TABLE 4 CLINICAL TYPOLOGICAL CLASSIFICATION OF HIGHER NERVOUS ACTIVITY (JORDANIA)

	Strong, unbalanced (excitable)	*Strong, balanced (lively)*	*Strong, balanced (inert)*	*Weak, unbalanced (inhibited)*
A Basic processes of higher nervous activity: 1 Excitation 2 Inhibition	Excitation prevails over inhibition	The two fundamental processes occur in equal proportions		Inhibition prevails over excitation
B Fundamental properties of nervous processes:	Satisfactory capacity for work	Good capacity for work		Rapid tiring while working; submits easily; lack of perseverance
1 Force	Perseverance in attaining a goal			
2 Equilibrium	Lack of self-control; no patience; excessive behaviour reactions; lack of movements and gestures	Control and self-discipline	Meticulousness and excessive caution in all action	Dominance of inhibition
3 Mobility	Rapid transition from a state of rest to excitation	Rapid adjustment to the environment, and to new circumstances	Slow adjustment to the environment, particularly new ones; slow actions	Indifference to outside events
C The state of higher nervous activity at different times of life:		Moderate participation in all life happenings		
1 Initial period (first memories)	Takes part in and leads noisy games; wants to lead; shows initiative	Lively participation in the events of childhood		Tendency to remain outside noisy games; whining

2 Period of sexual maturation	Tendency to break away from parental protection			Unwarranted sensitivity; whining; easily influenced by friends
3 Period of sexual maturity		Self-mastery in familial and daily relations		
4 Menopause	Rapid manifestation of the failure of ovarian function	Good tolerance of the failure of ovarian function		Ill-defined manifestations of failure of ovarian function
D At different times in life:				
1 Capacity for work and reserve of strength	Initiative; great perseverance in attaining a goal	Hard worker; large energy reserve		Frequent refusal to do extra work; lack of initiative
2 Behaviour in the face of danger	Perseverance in overcoming obstacles	Rapid assessment of a situation before acting	Slow assessment of a situation before taking a decision	No perseverance; tends to avoid decisions in vital situations
3 Behaviour in a medical establishment	Conflicts with staff; refusal of treatment	Refusal of treatment	Complete confidence in all exigencies in hospital	Excessive fears preceding choice of treatment
Alcohol	Rapid excitation	Moderate excitation		Debilitating effect with weakness of the two processes
Ether Bromides	Slow in going to sleep Momentary balance of fundamental nervous processes	Rapid sleep		Oppression of the nervous state
Caffeine	Excitation increased			When the dose is diminished, excitatory functions increase

inadequacy is, today, generally recognized. We may, however, emphasize the distance between the use of such a summary classification and a comprehensive investigation. Yet, in the very midst of the detailed information to which attention is directed, one is struck by the static nature of the indices (for example, attentiveness, capacity for distraction); the vaguely defined idea of objectivity underlying the method may also be noted. Despite the aridity of the reported results, the impression remains that the Russian system of classification does contain the possibility of predicting the quality of the confinement, or at least behaviour during confinement.

Outside the frame of reference of preparation

Here we shall find some studies to which we have already referred. These will serve to remind us of various procedures, all of which contributed to the isolation of determining 'factors' in childbirth.

A first group of studies is concerned with the investigation of the women's *attitudes* and *feelings* by means of questionnaires or interviews. Ferreira (54) uses 'negative maternal attitude' as a variable. Winokur and Werboff (156) use an eight-point questionnaire including, in particular, the following:

Was this pregnancy expected?
Do you wish, at the moment, to have a child?
Did you wish to have a child at the beginning of your pregnancy?
Make a two-sentence statement of how you feel about having a child.

Newton (115) studies 'maternal emotions'. She wonders whether women's 'feelings' towards menstruation, pregnancy, etc. are related to other physical, psychological, or social phenomena. She finds relationships between such 'feelings' and the dose of drugs received during confinement. It would appear to follow that the feelings expressed by expectant mothers on a number of crucial matters foreshadow the quality of their confinement.

Newton's method is based upon the hypothesis that 'human emotions can be studied by statistical methods'. Desires, fears, etc. are recorded and classified by a judge unacquainted with the subjects, on the basis of interview records.

The main feature of this type of research is that objectivity is achieved by the strict classification of responses and the absence of interpretation. It is obvious, however, that feelings, desires, and fears are not as simple as this. In particular, unconscious drives or defences play their part in the expression of positive and negative 'emotions'. The manifest content can, nevertheless, be used, with its underlying significance indicated 'in parentheses'. This method may facilitate the establishment of relationships among data which might at first appear quite heterogeneous, but it soon comes up against the need for explanatory hypotheses which it cannot provide.

A second approach uses psychometric methods. Davids *et al.* (41) have followed this course with a battery of tests of which they mention only two, the Wechsler Scale and the Taylor Manifest Anxiety Scale. It is, of course, not without interest to seek possible correlations between results obtained with such tests and data collected on childbirth. But once again, this does not lead to an explanatory hypothesis.

On the other hand, other tests have an intrinsic theoretical basis, which enables hypotheses concerning *determining* factors of childbirth to be formulated. Such tests have been used in another category of research aiming at the classification of the women themselves; thus Scott and Thompson (144) have attempted to relate the psychological state of primiparae in the sixth month of pregnancy to the duration and course of labour. They divided the women into stable, unstable, and intermediate on the basis of *contemporary* clinical data. According to these authors there is a positive relationship between 'instability' (behind which lies latent anxiety) and difficulties in labour such as long duration, termination, etc.

INVESTIGATIONS NOT CENTRED UPON CONFINEMENT

Klein, Potter, and Dyk (83), to whom we have already referred, have studied anxiety during pregnancy and confinement. They advance no preliminary hypothesis and proceed straight away to accumulate data by means of semi-directive interviews (i.e. interviews involving the systematic exploration of a certain number of variables). As far as the global classification of the women is concerned, the authors also adopt the bipolar dimension stable-unstable, which they define as follows:

> stable women are free of neurotic symptoms, mature, and adjusted to their conditions of living even if these are strenuous;
> unstable women tend to be dependent and immature, and to show neurotic symptoms.

61

In addition, Klein, Potter, and Dyk made a systematic record of:

emotional attitudes, fears, desires, etc. (especially with respect to the child);

objective information concerning the sociocultural level, antecedents, the circumstances surrounding conception, etc.;

symptoms during pregnancy.

We have already noted (p. 52) the variables they used to establish relevant relationships (good or bad confinement, positive or negative psychological reaction).

We summarize below the main conclusions of these authors, bearing in mind that their work was not centred primarily upon confinement:

(a) Forms of behaviour during pregnancy and confinement do not always coincide.

(b) The intensity of the desire for children is not a valid indication for a successful confinement.

(c) A good confinement is not necessarily accompanied by a positive psychological reaction.

(d) Stable women show a positive psychological reaction whether labour is good or bad.

(e) Unstable women show a positive psychological reaction only if labour is good.

(f) Women who show many symptoms during pregnancy are just as likely as others to have a satisfactory confinement both physiologically and psychologically.

(g) All women retain a traumatic memory of their delivery.

(h) As far as anxiety is concerned, there is a correspondence between pregnancy and confinement.

(i) There is no obvious relationship between the duration of labour and the size of the baby, the age of the mother, or her rejection of the child.

The authors conclude that a great many variables play a part in confinement (although it is defined in this study, as we have seen, in terms of two variables only). These contributing variables include:

character structure and emotional make-up

attitude towards pregnancy

emotional preparation and confidence in the hospital

pharmacology and analgesia

physical and physiological structure.

The authors give no guide to the relative importance or interrelation of these factors. They advance the hypothesis that, in certain cases, there is such a close connexion between the physiological process of labour and the subject's basic constitution that emotional factors have no noticeable effect upon the mechanism of labour.

This investigation represents a very fruitful pilot study, the defects of which (as admitted by the authors themselves) derive from a certain vagueness in the terms used, both to describe the subjects (stable or unstable), and to define their feelings (these are not always clearly specified as conscious or unconscious) and the quality of the confinement (what, for instance, is a 'good' psychological reaction?).

Despite these shortcomings, this study raises in a striking way fundamental problems related to the assembling of 'factors' at very different levels. For one ought to know how interdependent such factors are, or at least how they combine (the problem of quantification).

This study by Klein, Potter, and Dyk included confinement among its concerns. The investigations to which we now turn our attention are not directly concerned with confinement, and are mentioned only in so far as they may provide us with valuable suggestions through their hypotheses and especially through the classification of their subjects.

The work of Bibring *et al.* (13, 14, 15) has several times been referred to. Bibring's detailed approach to the crisis of pregnancy, its basic meaning, the changes in the ego and the outside world to which it leads, and the maturing aspect of the experience, has been, for us, a constant source of inspiration. Methodologically, his approach is inspired by psychoanalytic thinking and he is concerned with a small sample of women whom he studied in great depth. In the next chapter an account will be given of our attempts to interpret our own limited data in psychoanalytic terms, and our lack of success.

Pavenstedt (124) starts from the hypothesis that immature mothers will have children whose development is disturbed as compared with that of children of mature mothers. This hypothesis can be subdivided and leads to two lines of investigation:

The degree of maturity and integration of children at the age of six may be compared with the judgement originally made concerning

63

the maturity of their mothers. This comparison is made by means of a statistical analysis of the relationship between personality variables of mother and child.

Disturbances in the child's development may be studied in relation to the mother's personality structure. This requires a mainly clinical approach to the mother-child relationship.

This division of the initial hypothesis is of interest to us because it suggests a corresponding division for our study on childbirth. On the one hand, we may compare personality variables with the objective variables of confinement; on the other hand, we may make a global clinical study of confinement in the light of the information available on the woman's personality and on the structure of interpersonal relationships within the labour ward, which together lead to a certain style of initial mother-child relationship and a certain type of behaviour of the newborn.

Pavenstedt defines maturity as a genetic-dynamic concept indicating the 'flexibility with which ego functions mediate between the unconscious impulses and reality to obtain optimum gratification for the individual without arousing undue anxiety or incurring serious guilt feelings, so that energy becomes available for relationships, activities, interests and creativeness'.

Pavenstedt then gives a list of traits characteristic of each of three groups of women:

Group A – the relatively more mature mothers

This group includes women whose development has been smooth in an affectionate, stable environment; who have passed from one stage of development to the next at approximately the average age, having resolved the major conflicts of the previous period; who have had the usual succession of relationships and have become emancipated from their parents, leaving them little dependent on the older generation yet able to turn to them for advice. They are women whose feminine identification and capacity for relating closely to the important people in their lives have led to a marriage based on reason, tenderness, and sexual compatibility; whose desire it is to have a home and children, with moderate ambitions to improve their situation in life but without fixed notions of what they wish their children to be; whose child-rearing concepts have been absorbed from their mothers, aunts, older sisters, and friends, so that they feel secure about raising children; whose organization, evidenced in the past by competence, by adequate performance at school and at work, will now be evident in sound planning for their home and their husband's comfort; whose sense of identity and of security are such that they need not resort to primitive defences; who may respond to change under stress with transitory symptoms and regressive tendencies but who will recover their psychic equilibrium in due time; who are not given to impulsive outbursts or to marked mood swings; whose conscience is sufficiently unburdened to allow them to enjoy their family life without feeling that they are sacrificing themselves. Finally, they relate to the interviewers with some reserve at first but with a growing sense of trust.

Group B – the middle group

The intermediate group includes women who have developed a firm defensive structure which enables them to make an adequate adaptation to their situation in life; who may be obliged to remain in or return to situations very similar – geographically and socio-economically – to their childhood background because a change constitutes a threat from which they withdraw (with adequate rationalizations); whose relationships to people may be markedly ambivalent; whose failure to resolve their dependency needs may be expressed by having to remain close to their families or, in contrast, by exaggerated attitudes and gestures of independence and self-sufficiency; whose need to control their own feelings, their relationships, their interviews with us, our contacts with their husbands, etc., is constantly in the forefront; in whom anxiety is held in abeyance but may become quite evident at times to the interviewer; who may suffer from a character neurosis or from various neurotic symptoms (such as phobias, conversion symptoms, psychosomatic symptoms, emotional lability) that are not so severe as to interfere seriously with their circumscribed life situation; who tend to have quite definite and fixed ideas about child-rearing, often on the side of punishment and control; whose sexual identity is not altogether clear; who tend to feel superior to or defensive about their husbands; for whom marriage and motherhood are states that they accept, but with varying degrees of trepidation; who express hesitation and doubt about whether they are really pregnant during the first trimester; whose anxiety connected with sex and procreation may be quite severe and often controlled by infantile defences; whose fantasy life remains primitive so that they have to restrict their lives to protect themselves against a world conceived of as crudely instinctual (although most of this will be largely inhibited from coming into consciousness). Their personalities are not well integrated, frequently there is a definite split into good and bad. They need to bolster their self-esteem by praise gathered here and there for relative achievements; the self-image is usually impaired; there is often a restless need for activity,

65

work – with little time, for example, for reflection, reading, or handwork; there is little evidence of sublimation. Mood swings may be prominent. During interviews, these women are often very guarded and loath to reveal themselves but gradually become more communicative as we succeed in meeting their dependent needs without threatening their independence.

Group C – the most immature group

This group includes women who may have been seriously traumatized in the course of their development – by losses, separations, broken homes, serious pathology in a parent, prolonged illness, etc. They may show or have shown evidence of psychopathic trends, severe neurosis, psychosomatic illness, extreme mood swings, or of borderline psychotic conflicts and defences beneath a brittle surface adjustment; that is, women whose adaptive functioning is *not* well maintained. They may have ill-defined ego boundaries, and a poorly established sense of identity, with confused sexual identity. Women whose relationships have been stormy, shallow, suspicious, competitive, or otherwise unrewarding, whose achievements at school and work were far below their potentialities, will be included in this group. Their poor self-control often leads to impulsive acting-out followed by feelings of guilt and self-reproach or projections onto others. As a result of deprivation, most of them will remain extremely demanding and dependent and will be unwilling and unable to enter into marriage or to contemplate the arrival of an offspring with the necessary selflessness; they will feel abused. Their homes and lives and their communications to us will lack organization and logic; an attempt may be made at control by means of rigid formulae or routines. Since change to this group is so threatening, there will be, in general, a tendency to sameness, with stereotypy as an extreme or, on the other hand, an impulsive change in flight. Illusory omnipotence or other magical devices may be resorted to so that the subject's ability to test reality becomes precarious.

There is no need to emphasize, with the author, the heterogeneous character of these observations and the tentative meaning of the concept of maturity. Before we see what kind of order Pavenstedt introduces into these data, one of her conclusions calls for special comment here: *the ease and smoothness of the confinement are unrelated to the maturity (as here defined) of the parturient woman's personality.* In fact, some of the most immature mothers have the easiest confinements, and vice versa, although this is not consistently so. This does not mean that character structure has no bearing upon confinement, but that *the factors involved are other than maturity.*

Among the other determining factors, Pavenstedt draws attention to the particular relationship of the woman with the obstetrician, the presence of specific conflicts (relating to the body-image, the fact of being pregnant, etc.), the presence of certain constellations of character traits (for example, narcissistic vulnerability with strong and effective control of vital situations), and certain obstetrical factors such as the state of the cervix at the onset of labour.

All these data are important in that they indicate *at what level* discrimination with regard to the predisposing factors has to be made if these are to have any chance of correlating with the *diverse* variables of childbirth. A global classification of the women, even a finely discriminative one, is not sufficient. The possibility of segmental studies, referring back to certain areas of the personality or life-history of the subject, must be retained.

In an intermediate report (123), Pavenstedt and her colleagues provide some interesting models of possible partial scoring. For a better evaluation of the mother's personality they use scales of isolated psychological variables. Their summation would give a *total score* or even a *rank* for each mother. It will presently be seen how, at a less ambitious level (since our material is not so rich), we have tried to solve simultaneously the problem of an inventory of past or present personal data and that of their partial or total summation, which is essential if such data are to be related to aspects of childbirth.

The maternal character variables used by Pavenstedt and her colleagues are as follows:

External functioning
pathological symptoms:

> psychosomatic
> neurotic
> psychopathic
> borderline psychotic.

capacity for compromise formation (the ability to modify inner needs or ideals in favour of what appears to be the best solution in reality):

> capacity for recovery from the impact of stress
> capacity to experience genuine pleasure and happiness
> capacity to modify the environment

67

capacity for relationships
general effectiveness.

Intrapsychic functioning
degree of integration (body-image is too often disturbed during
pregnancy to serve as a reliable variable)
defence mechanisms
self-appraisal (the degree to which the subject can see herself realisti-
cally)
strength of fixation
feminine identification
anxiety
guilt feelings
masochism.

The authors emphasize the methodological difficulty involved in the
use of such variables. Clearly, there must be a sufficient degree of
agreement among several judges, and this level of agreement is more
difficult to attain, the less 'typical' the woman is.

This rapid review of the methods employed in the collection and
organization of data hypothetically appearing as determining factors
of confinement will help the reader to appreciate more clearly not
only the nature but also the limitation of the tools used in the present
research and described later. These limitations were imposed by the
type and abundance of the material obtained. But, like Pavenstedt
(123, 124), we were anxious to develop as far as possible a convenient
instrument which might even be simplified and, as such, usable by
non-specialists (obstetricians or general practitioners) for the detec-
tion of expectant mothers who, from the beginning, pose a problem
in prognosis.

SUMMARY

This chapter, which consists largely of an analytical review of the
literature, considers the researches conducted and the methods used
to collect and organize physiological and psychological data thought
to be related to possible 'factors influencing childbirth'.

It raises the following important questions and examines the solutions that have been proposed:

What aspects of childbirth should be observed and recorded?

How can the problem of pain and the problem of behaviour be brought together?

What aspects (nervous type or character type, anxiety, maturity, etc.) should be singled out for classifying the women and for establishing relationships between such a classification and records of confinements?

It also indicates the limitations of the tools used, and gives some idea of the methodological difficulties involved in this type of research, such as the difficulty of bringing together observations in different areas and at different levels, and of developing a simple and usable instrument that will not only provide a basis for classification, but also enable correlations to be established and predictions made.

G. GAYLE STEPHENS, M.D.
3232 East Pine
Wichita, Kansas 67208

CHAPTER 4

The Research

As soon as the theoretical bases of our research had been determined, we decided that our study should be confined to a sample of *married, primiparous, French* women, whether prepared for childbirth or not. The research sample therefore consists of only a small number of those women who attended the maternity department for prenatal examination.

The parturient women who fulfilled the necessary conditions were referred directly to the investigators by the consulting physician after their first gynaecological examination. At the first interview, which was conducted in a medical setting, the subjects were informed that a psychological investigation was being carried out, and another appointment was made. Most of the women accepted this in good spirit, only two women out of 250 objecting to the follow-up of the interviews.

This arrangement depended upon a pre-existing agreement between the medical staff and the research team, which was composed of psychiatrists, psychoanalysts, and psychologists. The introduction of such a team into a maternity department raised some minor difficulties of two kinds: those connected with its being a psychological team and those connected with its being a research team.

To start with, our interests as members of a psychological team were very different from those of the gynaeco-obstetrical team. The psychological approach to the pregnant woman and the conditions of confinement, which was our main objective, was only a secondary aspect of the work of the obstetricians and midwives, and the mistrust with which medical practitioners are in the habit of regarding psychologists is well known. We had, therefore, to break down this mistrust in order that we might be accepted and might obtain the cooperation of the whole department, since the work could not proceed otherwise.

Again, as members of a research team, we were inevitably regarded as a parasitic entity, doing work from which no hospital department could gain any immediate benefit. It was in order to overcome this impression of uselessness, which could have been harmful to us, that we endeavoured to meet the needs of the department with respect to the psychosomatic problems of some of the women, and the feelings of mutual assistance that were thus created facilitated our work. Thus our investigation represents one of the rare examples of interdisciplinary research in a department of a French general hospital.

DATA USED IN THE INVESTIGATION

The research data comprise, on the one hand, psychological information collected during pregnancy, and, on the other hand, observations concerning confinement.

Psychological data collected during pregnancy

We decided to see the women three times, at three definite points during their pregnancy, for an interview lasting on average one hour.

The first interview was before the third month of pregnancy; at this point, the baby is not yet physically perceived by the mother as an entity distinct from herself. The second interview was immediately after the first movements of the baby, thus usually during the fourth month, at that critical point at which the mother becomes aware of an existence independent of and yet fundamentally dependent upon her own. The third and last interview was at the end of the eighth month of pregnancy, near to the confinement. It enabled us to find out how the women prepared by the PPM had experienced this preparation, and how much benefit they had derived from it; and to appreciate, in all the women, the conscious or unconscious anxiety exacerbated or repressed during this pre-confinement period.

The purpose of these interviews was twofold: first, to collect as many data as possible on the woman's personal history; and, second, to apprehend, through these data, her deep-lying movitations, the expression of her anxieties, her mechanisms of defence, and the structure of her personality.

At the beginning of the research, we examined a certain number of women who have not been included in the experimental sample. This pilot study enabled us to refine our method of investigation and resulted in our drawing up interview guidelines, which specified the areas

71

that were to be systematically explored (see the guidelines at the end of the present chapter, pp. 83-85).

The function of these guidelines was simply to define a minimum body of information to be obtained from all subjects, and they were in no way intended as a rigid framework limiting psychological investigation. Although we had to obtain the same kind of information on a number of questions from all subjects, in order that the data could readily be standardized, we also regarded it as essential that the women observed should feel free to express themselves. Each woman had to be left free to develop in her own way the themes suggested, to vary the emphasis given, and to enlarge upon any problems that seemed to be important for her. This freedom was encouraged by the complete neutrality of the observer.

The method of semi-directive interview that we had decided to adopt appeared to be the procedure most appropriate to our research aims. In so far as it is hoped to reach the deep-lying personality, genuinely non-directive contact is no doubt more productive; but within the limits of three interviews, which had had to be agreed, the material that could have been collected in this way would have been too fragmentary and too varied from one woman to another for a general interpretation to have been possible. Conversely, strictly objective methods, such as those employing questionnaires, would have facilitated the collection of homogeneous and easily quantifiable material, but would have limited the range of this material and, in particular, would have decreased its meaningfulness.

The method chosen has thus indisputable advantages, but the difficulties that it involves should not be ignored. The most serious difficulty arises from the fact that the semi-directive method is also semi-interpretative. It requires the interviewer to provide orientation without ever suggesting anything, and to be continually selecting, from among the observations made by the subject, those which it is useful to encourage her to develop. In this flexible conduct of the interview one must be able to go beyond the subject's rationalizations in order to overcome the ambiguity of her responses. This attempt to achieve immediate understanding and interpretation is pursued during a dialogue between two people, which obviously cannot be repeated, with all its nuances, and which also inevitably involves an element of subjectivity. We found, however, that when the interviews were entrusted to two clinicians of very different personalities, they finally reached essential agreement on the way in which the interview should be conducted and the information recorded. This method can obviously be used only by a good clinician, capable of making a rapid provisional psychological diagnosis, and modifying his attitude to the patient and orienting his relation to her accordingly. He must also be sufficiently trained in psychoanalysis to be able to distinguish deep from superficial aspects, and to discern the defence mechanisms through which the personality of the subject is expressed.

It thus appears that the method selected essentially combines the advantages of the clinical method and the so-called objective methods. It takes over from the clinical method the possibility of orienting the interview towards specific areas of information, while at the same time respecting the individuality of the subject's reactions and psychological structure; and, from the objective methods, the concern with obtaining homogeneous and quantifiable data. It represents, in fact, a compromise between two methodological requirements often regarded as incompatible: that of an 'understanding' approach to psychological questions and that of an 'objective' procedure. Without fully meeting either of these requirements, the method endeavours to avoid sacrificing one to the other. In order that the reader may more fully understand the *modus operandi* and appreciate the resources and limitations of our method, three case-histories chosen from the sample studied are presented in Appendix I, and the 'interview guides' may be consulted at the end of this chapter.

In addition to the interviews, a number of psychological tests were used. These were not applied systematically to all the women in the sample. Instead, different tests were given to different sub-samples of women. This psychometric material is intended to form the basis of cross-sectional studies which will be published later. The following tests were used:

MMPI
Z test
Body-sway test (test of suggestibility)
Adaptation of the Taylor Manifest Anxiety Scale.

Data collected during confinement

If the aims of the investigation were to be achieved, it appeared indispensable to observe the women directly during their confinement. Systematic observations were therefore made by the psychiatrist in the team, who was present in the labour ward from the start of the confinement. These observations constituted the basic material, but, to supplement this information, the form filled in by the midwives at the time of the confinement was also used, as was the obstetrical record.

The observer was called when the woman was about three fingers dilated and remained present during the whole of labour, including delivery. He always tried to reconstruct as far as possible, by means of an interview with the parturient woman, what had occurred before his arrival, i.e. from the first signs of the onset of labour.

The presence of a psychiatric observer in the labour ward could not but raise definite and sometimes very difficult problems, essentially connected with the ambiguity of his position in relation to the midwives and the parturient women themselves. As far as the midwives and nurses were concerned, they sometimes regarded the observer as a useless character whose non-activity they found irritating in a situation which for them was one demanding, above all, action and efficiency. They might even, in extreme cases, regard him as an embarrassing witness, in so far as they might think that he was there to watch their work and pass judgement on their attitudes and behaviour with regard to the parturient women. As far as the latter themselves were concerned, they naturally expected some help from this doctor who stayed so long beside them for their special benefit. Thus a demanding attitude on the part of the woman towards the observer often developed. The observer, however, was supposed to remain an objective spectator. Nevertheless, it can readily be understood that, in the actual labour ward situation, the observer often found himself involved in an interpersonal complex which sometimes obliged him to depart from his neutrality. Whenever this happened, the problem arose as to the 'distance' it was best to adopt. In order that this material might be used in a general analysis the observer always took care to make a very detailed note of all these interpersonal occurrences, as also of such interventions by the various protagonists as might affect the situation in any way.

The material thus collected was quite complex and revealing, and included data at three different levels: obstetrical, behavioural, and psychological data.

The obstetrical data were provided by the medical record, and might be more detailed when the obstetrical facts were such as possibly

74

to have some influence on the behaviour or the psychological experience of the woman.

The basic behavioural data concerned motor behaviour – signs, screams or groans, spontaneous verbalizations, etc. Also included, for prepared women, was the way in which they applied the techniques learned during preparation – relaxation, breathing, and bearing down.

The more complex behavioural data implied a certain amount of psychological interpretation: they concerned the atmosphere of the labour ward, the general appearance presented by the woman, and the ways in which she interacted with the obstetrical staff. Also included here was the information obtained by the observer from talking with the woman (pain felt, anxiety expressed), and from noting her behaviour at the actual time of the birth and her immediate relation to the child.

This complex of data was supplemented by information collected in an interview two days after the confinement. This interview was conducted by a member of the team who already knew the woman from having had a previous interview with her, but who was not present during the confinement. This interview was intended:

(a) to complete the data provided by observation of the confinement, by asking the woman to give a retrospective account of her confinement, by stages;

(b) to obtain a subjective account from the woman of her experience during her confinement (painful or anxiety-laden); it was hoped that this account would enable a better interpretation to be made of the data derived from observation; and interesting discrepancies might also emerge between the woman's own account and the data obtained by observation;

(c) to obtain a subjective evaluation from the woman of the effects of the PPM, including a global estimate of its analgesic effect and a specific assessment of the role of the different elements in preparation (technique, information, and interpersonal support);

(d) to permit an evaluation of the relation of the woman to her baby at the time (attitude and behaviour with regard to breast-feeding, and plans for the future).

75

DESCRIPTION OF THE SAMPLE

As has already been stated, we had decided to study a sample of married primiparous women of French nationality. Our aim was to form two groups within this sample: a group of women prepared by the psychoprophylactic method as provided in the department, and a group of unprepared women. We had hoped to form two samples of equal size in order to facilitate statistical treatment, but it proved very difficult to find a sufficient number of unprepared women who fulfilled the requirements laid down. In fact, the majority of young primiparous women spontaneously choose to have preparation for childbirth. In France, to refuse to have preparation is to refuse a certain kind of up-to-dateness, and even young women who are unwilling to believe in, or do not feel that they are entitled to believe in, possible analgesia, show 'curiosity' or a desire to 'try the experiment' which, if it does not do them any good, at least will not do them any harm. Moreover, if any young women have an ambivalent attitude towards preparation, they will seek information when they first come to the department and cannot fail to hear the hospital and medical staff praising the method, and thus to have their motives for accepting it reinforced. It cannot, however, be said that the maternity department exercises any direct pressure on women in favour of the PPM, although the climate is favourable to the method. Thus, at the Hôpital Rothschild, only one woman out of five refuses preparation, which corresponds approximately to the average proportion noted in Parisian maternity wards over a period of several years. It therefore seems clear that refusal of preparation is much more uncommon than its acceptance (34).

Preparation for childbirth is practised as follows in the department. The women follow the routine of preparation from the seventh month of their pregnancy. They attend eight sessions, consisting of four sessions of theoretical instruction given by the doctors and four practical sessions given by the midwives.

The *theoretical instruction* includes:

(a) one lecture giving general information on the history of preparation for childbirth, some details of Pavlovian physiology, some observations on the problems of pain and psychological analgesia, and some principles of mental hygiene;

(b) one lecture on the anatomy and physiology of pregnancy, from conception to birth, and including some comments on physical hygiene and diet;

(c) one lecture on the course of confinement (before confinement, first signs of labour, admission to hospital, dilatation, taking up of the cervix, expulsion of the foetus, delivery of the placenta, possible obstetrical pathology);

(d) the last theoretical lecture, which is given only after the women have attended the whole of their practical training, consists of a general revision which is intended mainly as a kind of reassuring conversation with the women; the different stages in confinement are gone over again quickly, and the future mother-child relationship, in a mental health perspective, is briefly touched upon.

The *practical training* includes:

(a) revision of the main theoretical ideas, and instruction in relaxation technique (Jacobson's method);

(b) the learning of various respiratory rhythms adapted to the successive phases of dilatation, and relaxation exercises;

(c) relaxation exercises, breathing exercises, and the learning of respiratory and muscular movements for the moment of expulsion;

(d) revision of all the techniques learned.

These classes take place over a period of two months, with one session each week. The practical preparation in the department in which our research was carried out is sufficiently representative of the kind of preparation provided by hospitals in general. It begins rather late in pregnancy in order that it can be wholly included within the leave of absence allowed to working women who are having babies, two months before their confinement is due.

A general summary of the material collected during the research will now be given. In all, we compiled 204 case-histories of women who met the criteria for the sample. Some of these, however, remained incomplete and could not therefore be incorporated in the analysis. There were various reasons for their being incomplete. For some women, it was impossible to undertake all three interviews: for example, because of an interrupted pregnancy, or absence at the time of the appointment (through moving house, holidays, etc.), or illness, or failure to attend when asked, indicating reservations with regard to the research team. For other women, observations on their confinement were not obtained, either because they did not have their babies in the department, or because the observer was by chance unable to be present at the confinement. Thus a number of incomplete records had to be eliminated. The criteria according to which the final sample was selected were as follows:

The case-record had to include at least two interviews. In fact, some records with two interviews appeared to contain as much information as complete records. The first interview always had to be included because the record was opened on that occasion. When the second interview was missing, the psychologist had to obtain sufficient retrospective information during the third interview. When the third interview was missing, in most cases a substitute interview was obtained after the confinement, likewise seeking the necessary retrospective information.

The record had to furnish *in toto* sufficiently detailed information for the purposes of analysis, independently of the number of interviews. Thus it was necessary to discard some records in which the interviews had not yielded enough information, whether because of excessive reticence on the woman's part or because of genuinely low intelligence. These records may well have been just as interesting clinically as the others, but it seemed impossible to regard them as comparable. Among the records retained, the richness of the material varied quite considerably from one woman to another, and it was simply a question of fixing a level with regard to the quantity of the information that was available; above this level, records could be regarded as sufficiently homogeneous to lend themselves to an overall analysis.

Finally, the record had of course to include observations made during the confinement, since these were to form the basis of a number of variables, the analysis of which was one of the main purposes of the research.[1]

[1] The case-histories that lack an observer's report on the confinement could be used for a complementary research in which it would be sufficient, as far as confinement is concerned, to use the information provided by the obstetrical record and the midwives' report.

On the basis of these criteria, a *final sample* was selected consisting of 90 women prepared by the psychoprophylactic method and 26 unprepared women.

This final sample of 90 + 26 subjects is not, therefore, as we had originally intended, a random sample. The idea of a random sample is, moreover, one that must be treated with caution. In any case, we would not have obtained a random sample of all primiparous Parisian women, even if we had retained all the primiparae attending the maternity department of the Hôpital Rothschild. Such a sample would, in fact, have represented a particular population with very special characteristics, the population that attends the maternity department of the Hôpital Rothschild. It might be thought that the population of a hospital department is likely to be representative at least of the population belonging to a certain social class in one quarter of Paris. The maternity department of the Hôpital Rothschild, however, has been part of the health service for only seven years, before which it was the maternity department of a private Jewish foundation, and, as a result of this previous position, it has retained a traditional core of women patients who come from considerable distances to have their babies in the place where they themselves were born. Thus the population with which the present study is concerned includes a proportion (20 per cent) of Jewish women much higher than that in the population of Paris as a whole.

It will be obvious that the final sample of 90 + 26 women represents an even more specialized sample in view of the way in which it was selected. All the women who were retained according to the criteria laid down, as having complete records, were women who had agreed to give their time in order to provide the long interviews required. Their motives were various: a well-adjusted attitude of cooperation, pure self-satisfaction, pleasure at being retained as subjects in a scientific investigation, etc. Moreover, the interviews may have had a secondary cathartic effect which caused certain women of their own accord to seek further contacts with the psychologist, or to continue a kind of transference relationship with him after the end of their stay in hospital.

DEVELOPMENT OF METHODS OF ANALYSIS

As the investigation proceeded, we became familiar, through meetings for the purpose of coordination, with the data collected both from the interviews and from reports on the confinement, and we were, in consequence, better able to appreciate the kinds of information provided by these two levels of operation, and therefore to assess the practical possibilities they offered for establishing relationships. At the same time, a search of the literature provided us with a number of possible 'models' for this kind of operation (see preceding chapters). For about two years, these meetings enabled clinical material to be considered in relation to possible ways of classifying both women and confinements. The psychologist who had conducted the interviews read them out verbatim, interspersing his own comments on how they developed, on the impression the woman created, and on the kind of contact established. From this starting-point, we attempted to reconstruct the woman's personal history as fully as possible, emphasizing the main points and interpreting freely in psychoanalytic terms. After this, each member was free to make suggestions concerning the prognosis of the confinement, in respect of both obstetrical aspects and behavioural or interpersonal aspects. Then and only then did the person who had observed the confinement make his report. The discussion that followed made clear whether there was or was not 'agreement' between the psychological record and the confinement, and also the reasons why a prognosis was shown to be correct or incorrect.

As a result of these tentative efforts, several scoring systems previously used by other researchers seemed inadequate for the purpose in hand, on various grounds.

First, there was the question of the quantitative and qualitative significance of the material concerning confinements that the present research made available. In the conditions described, the construction of a grid for scoring the confinements (see next chapter), which made use of a good part of the available material, was relatively straightforward. But a further requirement was that the method used for handling the material that concerned the women should appear clinically to lend itself to an attempt to establish relationships with the different aspects of confinement.

When this empirical requirement and the average level of information available were borne in mind, the various reported systems appeared either too ambitious or not ambitious enough. In particular, those deriving directly from psychoanalysis seemed to be too ambitious. In addition to the fact that our material was too often inadequate, psychoanalytic theories of character are not easily applied to so-called 'normal' women. Furthermore, the 'crisis' nature of pregnancy makes this kind of assessment particularly difficult. On the other hand, the identification of items inspired by clinical psychoanalysis (preferred defence mechanisms, narcissism and body-image, superego and ego ideal), which could if necessary be quantified, seemed likely to be profitable. It was felt that such items might be found to form sub-groups particularly significant in relation to confinement. The level of information contained in the records, however, did not enable assessments to be made sufficiently frequently or reliably, and the necessary systematization was impossible.

Other rating systems seemed either not ambitious enough or simply not relevant. Non-psychoanalytic theories of character were not dynamic enough (although Le Senne's (96) theory, for example, is not without interest for understanding behaviour during confinement). The use of a global concept (such as equilibrium, stability, maturity, etc.), even if carefully elaborated, seemed unsatisfactory because of the crisis nature of the state of pregnancy. We have in mind, for example, the maturity scale developed by Pavenstedt and her colleagues (124) (the authors themselves remark upon its failure to predict confinements), or, at a simpler level, the Taylor Manifest Anxiety Scale (Davids *et al.*, 41). In the latter example we have an instance of a method with no structural reference, which uses a simple form of quantification of emotions, affects, and opinions, negative or positive. Despite the results achieved by such methods (cf. Chapter 3), they seemed too summary for the present purpose.

The literature thus failed to provide anything that appeared appropriate to the objectives and approach of our research. It was, however, essential to go beyond pure clinical intuition if there was to be any chance of clarifying our hypotheses, or at least of developing analytical tools which would enable us to state these hypotheses clearly and possibly to verify them. The practical necessity of a provisional synthesis of our data, in the absence of more precisely formulated hypotheses, led to the construction of the negativity grid, which is presented in the next chapter.

SUMMARY

Our research was carried out with married, primiparous French women who were observed before and during confinement in a Paris maternity department (the maternity department of the Hôpital Rothschild, head of department Dr P. Walter). One group of these women was prepared for childbirth by the psychoprophylactic method. They were prepared in four theoretical lectures (basic anatomical and physiological information, and mental hygiene of pregnancy and confinement) and four practical sessions (instruction in techniques of breathing, relaxing, and bearing down).

The research was made possible by the introduction into the hospital of a research team consisting mainly of psychiatrists. psychoanalysts, and psychologists. Two types of data were collected for each woman.

Before confinement, psychological data were obtained by means of semi-directive interviews. The first of these took place in every case before the third month of pregnancy, the second a little after the first movements of the baby, the third shortly before confinement (eighth month). These interviews were conducted according to a pre-established framework which indicated the kind of information to be obtained but allowed a high degree of clinical flexibility in the nature of the contact. In this way, an attempt was made to collect the maximum amount of information about the personality of the woman, her attitudes to pregnancy and motherhood, her present life, and any aspects of her past experience which might, in one way or another, have repercussions on her present experience. Particular attention was paid to the nature of the relations that developed, in the course of these interviews, between the clinician and his patient.

During the confinement itself, as detailed observations as possible were made by a psychiatrist who was present in the labour ward in the role of external observer with respect to the gynaecological-obstetrical staff. These observations, supplemented by the midwives' reports, were concerned with three kinds of data:

the behaviour of the parturient woman, recorded in as much detail and as objectively as possible;

more complex psychological data, noted in the first instance at a more interpretative level, concerning the experience of childbirth, relations with other people in the labour ward, pain suffered, etc.;

genuinely obstetrical data.

This information was expanded, and occasionally corrected, by a final interview that took place two or three days after confinement.

More than 200 women were studied in this way. By eliminating incomplete records and taking account of the criteria established for the selection of the sample, the investigators retained for the final analysis 90 women prepared by the PPM and 26 unprepared women. The relatively small number of the latter is explained by the fact that, in the maternity department concerned, preparation is offered to all pregnant women and only a minority refuse it. This clearly raises difficult questions of sampling and of the comparability of the two groups, prepared and unprepared. It seems very probable that, from the time that the groups were constituted, personality factors were operative which must be taken into account when the results are examined.

On the basis of the material thus obtained, two analytical tools were developed, by successive stages and after numerous syntheses of individual cases. These were the negativity grid, which summarizes the data derived from the interviews, and the confinement rating system, both of which are described in the next chapter.

GUIDE FOR FIRST INTERVIEW

1 *Civil status:*
   surname, first name, maiden name, age;
   profession, address, date of marriage;
   duration of pregnancy.

2 *Socio-economic status:*
   husband's occupation and wife's occupation;
   couple's budget, car, financial assistance.

3 *Information in connexion with the hospital:*
   reason for choice of hospital;
   impression from first gynaecological examination.

4 *Knowledge of childbirth and of preparation for childbirth:*
   level of information on childbirth (reading, TV, conversation);
   fears and fantasies concerning childbirth;
   instruction within the family – age at which this was given;
   attitude of family and friends, especially of mother, towards preparation for childbirth;
   attitude to pain;
   whether preparation was chosen and reason for choice;
   knowledge of preparation for childbirth, acceptance or deeply motivated refusal of analgesia.

5 *Attitude to future motherhood:*
baby wanted or coming too soon;
desire for or fantasies concerning abortion;
practice of contraception.

6 *Pregnancy:*
well-defined symptoms of onset of pregnancy;
awareness of pregnancy;
psychosomatic symptoms, psychological reaction at start of pregnancy;
attitude of husband and of the two families to the pregnancy.

7 *Family constellation:*
parents, grandparents, siblings (age, character, occupation, relations with subject).

8 *Personal history:*
(a) from birth to puberty:
      birth, psychomotor development;
      childhood illnesses;
      type of education;
      relations with mother, father (or substitutes), and siblings;
(b) puberty:
      knowledge about menstruation and womanhood;
      psychological and gynaecological experience of first period;
(c) life as a young woman:
      outline of sexual life, knowledge of sex, attitude to men;
      social and professional life (interests, orientation).

GUIDE FOR SECOND INTERVIEW

1 *Development of the pregnancy:*
psychosomatic symptoms, psychological reaction to pregnancy (narcissism, fear of childbirth, fantasies about childbirth);
personality changes.

2 *First movements of the foetus:*
circumstances, subjective aspects, fear of the child, sex desired;
plans for arrangements for the birth and the immediate future of the child.

3 *Family life:*
development of psychological relations with husband and relations with mother.

4 *Mother:*
   past gynaecological history, gynaecological pathology;
   instruction given by mother on sex.

5 *Subject's adult life:*
   level of independence with regard to parents;
   social life;
   sexual life before marriage – trauma of first sexual relations;
   disturbances in sexual life;
   dyspareunia (miscarriages, whether induced or not, frigidity, etc.);
   change in sexual life since pregnancy.

GUIDE FOR THIRD INTERVIEW

1 *Development of the pregnancy:*
   psychosomatic and gynaecological symptoms;
   psychological development (reality of the child).

2 *Reaction to preparation for childbirth:*
   theoretical lectures – how much learned, interest;
   practical sessions – sensory experience of relaxation and breathing;
   interpersonal relations with other women and with person preparing.

3 *Present fear of childbirth*

N.B. After every interview the clinician should make a careful note of the woman's bearing, attitudes, and appearance, and of the nature of the contact established, so as to be able to follow the development of transference during the interviews. He should also note his own counter-transference reactions.

If necessary, areas which have not been sufficiently clarified during the previous interviews are further discussed.

CHAPTER 5

Analytical Tools

The present chapter describes the main analytical tools used in the research. In the light of the two preceding chapters, it should be clear that these tools were not based upon elaborate hypotheses concerning the relations between confinement and the antecedent factors that condition it. They were intended simply to meet the needs of a provisional working synthesis, and represented no more than a basis from which more precise hypotheses might be arrived at. Two such tools were developed, concerning respectively the antecedent factors and the confinement itself. The following sections indicate the grounds on which these were felt to be justified and describe their actual content.

ANTECEDENT FACTORS AND THE NEGATIVITY GRID

We have seen how the coordinating meetings, at which the actual handling of the contents of the case-records and the various approaches recorded in the literature were brought together, led us to rule out these reported research methods as being either too ambitious or irrelevant to the question of childbirth. We therefore arrived at a provisional solution, which met three conditions:

it made maximum use of the material in the case-histories;
it was quantifiable;
it did not involve too precisely framed hypotheses.

This solution is represented by the negativity grid, the content of which will be described in detail later. Suffice it here to say that it fulfils three aims.

The first is that it includes as much as possible of the information in the case-histories through a twofold system of tabulation, by chronology and by area. To begin with, therefore, the grid is simply a two-way table providing a detailed and systematic analysis of every case-history and *an easy way of recording critical events in time and in different areas of psychological reality.*

The second aim introduces a working hypothesis: *the choice of the negative.*

Clinical experience shows that, with every woman, especially during pregnancy, it is easier to perceive 'what is wrong' than 'what is right'. Indeed, the effectiveness of the integration of past conflicts and the strength and dynamic force of the ego are very difficult to assess in view of the widespread reactivation that takes place during the *state of crisis*. It is easier simply to record the negative factors that appear in the case-history, whether these are past or present events of a highly traumatic kind (such as a serious illness or the loss of a relative) or ordinary events that are mentioned during the interview in a context which suggests that they reflect some distortion (e.g. the birth of a brother, backwardness at school, etc.). It is scarcely necessary to mention the *a priori* methodological position implied here or the confused and heterogeneous nature of its referents. The absence of all negative signs from a case-history may indicate a certain attitude on the woman's part during the interviews, and the defences that such an attitude expresses, as well as the absence of conscious awareness of any developmental distortion or of any conflict. Thus an abstract norm emerges: that of a woman who, in the limiting case, has never known any conflicts, frustrations, or anxieties, and has never even had to make any efforts at adjustment.

The application of the principle of negativity in practice involves a selection from the material available such that only that which can be regarded as representing a factor or index of maladjustment or a possible source of anxiety is retained. It should also be remarked that the circumstances in which they were examined made the women in general emphasize their present or past difficulties rather than any positive aspects of their lives.

Once the principle of selection of the negative is accepted, there still remains the problem of defining, for each cell in the table, the criterion for the inclusion of possible items. An example will be given later of such criteria. But it can be appreciated that, from a practical point of view, the problems connected with the establishing of criteria for the inclusion of items in any cell, and the differences in criteria for different cells, are very pressing ones. What connexion is there between the criteria for the inclusion of negative items in the somatic pathology area, and those for the inclusion of items in the area of family relations or economic difficulties? This brings us to the third aim of the grid, to provide an orientation for this seemingly arbitrary collection of negative signs.

The need to define a criterion of negativity for each cell, instead of simply including in it all relevant negative items, follows from the principle that *the possible negative items in each cell should be of equal weight*. This means that one should be able to add them together to give an overall or *general index of negativity*, which might be considered as representing the anxiety potential of each woman. This index might then be used to facilitate a comparison and a convenient classification of the women. Its relationships with types of confinement could be investigated; and a positive relationship might then appear.

The concept that the entries in each cell of the table might be subject to simple summation confronts us in acute form with the problem of the total number of factors, of the breakdown of the material into chronological periods or psychological areas. This problem is closely associated with that of defining the criterion for inclusion in each cell separately. Indeed, it is clear that if the grid is handled by summing the items grouped in the different areas and periods, then the number of items included in each area, and their possible recurrence in the different time-divisions, will determine the relative importance of this area in the grand total. An area that includes profuse and detailed information, highly differentiated, will carry more weight than an area that comprises scanty information about a small number of variables which do not differentiate effectively.

It follows, therefore, that the relative weighting of the areas and periods, like the definition of the criterion of negativity for the entries in each cell, must be determined empirically on the basis of clinical experience. As will be shown later, the development of the grid proceeded by a series of tentative steps towards a kind of compromise between two interdependent requirements: to preserve for the grid its function as a systematic and comprehensive inventory of negative items; and to slant it in the direction of emphasizing those factors which, on clinical grounds, appeared *a priori* more likely to be relevant to predicting the quality of a confinement. For example, there is the course of feminine identification in all its aspects, which, because of its association with the problems of childbirth, should have a chance of being reflected in a large number of cells with relatively easy criteria for inclusion.

The definition of these thresholds or criteria for inclusion entails two kinds of norm: an ideal norm, according to which every item with negative indications would be included; and a statistical norm, to act as a filter to the ideal norm, for certain items that are undeniably negative but occur too frequently and are too common in our culture (for example, mild dysmenorrhoea or various financial difficulties) should not be recorded lest they adversely affect the discriminating power of the corresponding cells.

It must, accordingly, be emphasized that, in the last resort, the inclusion of any item as negative inevitably involves *interpretation*. The interpretation here, however, is of separate items and is consequently easier and less arbitrary than a more global interpretation. Further, interpretation is involved only in the case of items which are not manifestly traumatic, since these latter are included by definition.

These problems concerning the construction of the grid will presently become clear, when the actual grid is presented in its two successive forms.

It should be stressed, finally, that the grid must remain a very flexible instrument, which can be used both at the level of the global index of negativity and, more especially, at the level of the partial indices concerning areas or periods, so that the relationships of these indices with both the global and the partial indices of confinement may be studied.

DEVELOPMENT OF THE NEGATIVITY GRID

To illustrate the way in which the grid was evolved, as a compromise between several aims, its two successive forms will be described. Presented first is a preliminary version of the grid, which preceded its final and present form.

The first form of the grid was used in a pilot study, the results of which have already been published (35). The aims of this pilot study were:

to provide preliminary verification of our hypothesis of a relationship between 'total negativity' and quality of confinement, and thus to test the predictive value of the negativity grid;

to show the relative predictive value of the various aspects of negativity, and, on the basis of these findings, possibly to alter the weighting assigned in order to increase the global predictive value of the instrument.

The preliminary form of the grid is described briefly below, so that the reader may follow the changes that were introduced subsequently in the development of the final form.

FIRST FORM OF THE NEGATIVITY GRID

I AREAS OF NEGATIVITY

A *Individual pathology*
(a) traumatic experiences: surgical operations, physical accidents;
(b) general pathology: serious illnesses, chronic pathology;
(c) psychopathology, including neurotic tandencies;
(d) developmental difficulties in early childhood;
(e) psychosomatic symptoms during pregnancy.

B *Womanhood*
(a) personal gynaecological pathology;
(b) disturbances of the menstrual cycle: amenorrhoea, dysmenorrhoea;
(c) disturbances of psychosexual development, rejection of womanhood or motherhood, frigidity, etc.;
(d) failure in sex role: breaking off of love affair, trouble between couple.

C *Negativity relating to husband*
(a) traumatic experiences: death, accidents, etc.;
(b) general pathology;
(c) psychopathology and neurotic tendencies;
(d) interpersonal difficulties: conflicts, misunderstandings;
(e) difficulties in social adjustment experienced by the couple.

D *Negativity relating to mother*
(a) traumatic experiences: death, accidents, etc.;
(b) general pathology;
(c) gynaecological-obstetrical pathology;
(d) psychopathology and neurotic tendencies;
(e) interpersonal difficulties: maternal inadequacy, conflicts, etc.

E *Negativity relating to father*
(a) traumatic experiences: death, accidents, etc.
(b) general pathology (including all forms of pathology);
(c) interpersonal difficulties: paternal inadequacy, conflicts, etc.

F *Negativity relating to siblings*
(a) traumatic experiences: death, accidents, etc.
(b) general pathology (including all forms of pathology);
(c) interpersonal difficulties: conflicts, misunderstandings, etc.

G *Negativity relating to family background*
(a) traumatic experiences concerning members of family not already mentioned;
(b) disturbances of family structure: broken home, absence of parents, separation from family;
(c) interpersonal difficulties: conflicts, misunderstandings, etc., concerning members of family not already mentioned.

H *Social adjustment*
(a) traumatic experiences, essentially connected with the war;
(b) difficulties at school and at work;
(c) interpersonal difficulties concerning friends, colleagues, etc.
(d) financial difficulties.

II CHRONOLOGICAL PERIODS

Clear distinctions were made between the following periods:

> prenatal
> natal
> early childhood (from birth to six years)
> childhood (up to puberty)
> adolescence
> adult life before marriage
> marriage (considered as a critical event)
> conjugal life before pregnancy
> first period of pregnancy (up to the first movements of the foetus)
> second period of pregnancy (from the first movements of the foetus up to about the seventh month)
> third period of pregnancy (pre-confinement – eighth and ninth months).

It will be seen that the chronological periods were thus numerous and unequal in length, involving both extended periods and critical moments in time (e.g. birth, puberty).

The procedure followed was to pick out from the case-histories all the negativity items included in the grid and enter a cross in the appropriate cell for the area (or sub-area) and period, as the case might be. When any such negative item appeared of special importance, it was marked by a cross with a circle round it, and was given extra weight in the final addition which yielded the global index of negativity (one point was given for a cross and three points for a circled cross). Sixty case-histories were analysed with this first form of the negativity grid, 40 of women prepared by the psychoprophylactic method and 20 of unprepared women. For each of these 60 women, the global index of negativity was correlated with the global index of quality of confinement obtained by the confinement grid described later. The resulting correlation coefficient was 0·46, which appears to confirm the working hypothesis in a satisfactory manner. In addition, the pilot sample was divided into two subgroups on the basis of the failure or success of the confinement ('good' or 'poor' confinements, according to the global confinement index), and the results were examined to see which of the negativity items appeared more frequently in the 'poor' than in the 'good' group. It was thus possible to assess the relative predictive value of the different negativity items.

At this stage in the research, there appeared to be two alternative ways of developing the final form of the grid. We could concentrate upon making it an instrument to predict the quality of confinements, in which case only those items would be retained that occurred more frequently in poor than in good confinements. Alternatively, the grid might be allowed to retain its function as a systematic and comprehensive inventory of possible negative items at the expense of its predictive efficiency. This problem has already been mentioned. In fact, we decided to compromise: as far as possible, we attempted to attach more weight to the items that appeared most closely related to the failure of the confinement and, conversely, to attach less importance to the items that had little or no predictive value; but, at the same time, we sought to keep intact the overall structure of the grid, therefore most of the items were retained.

The majority of the changes were introduced for an essentially practical purpose – to make the tool simpler to use and more reliable. They consisted in regrouping items within areas or reassigning items to different areas, thus avoiding inconvenient overlapping between areas; and in altering some of the principles of scoring, by eliminating ambiguities or unnecessary complexities, or by modifying the actual criteria for scoring.

Thus the final form of the grid was both more logically constituted and simpler to operate. With regard to the predictive value of the revised instrument, we again calculated the correlation between global negativity index and quality of confinement, on the same sample as before, but using the new scoring criteria for negativity: a coefficient of the same order as before was obtained. Thus the compromise solution adopted meant that the revision of the grid did not add anything to its power to predict the quality of confinements. It did, however, substantially improve the formal properties of the instrument and probably also, by this very fact, its quality as a measuring instrument.

FINAL FORM OF THE GRID

STRUCTURE OF THE GRID

The general structure of the grid is that of a two-way table, one dimension representing *areas*, the other *chronological periods*. Each item is located in terms of this double system of reference. The grid is divided into two main parts corresponding to two major chronological divisions:

negativity in previous personal history;
negativity during pregnancy.

In the first part, three periods are distinguished:

childhood;
puberty and adolescence;
adulthood.

In the second part, two periods are distinguished:

up to the first movements of the child;
after the first movements of the child.

Each part includes the following areas and sub-areas:

I NEGATIVITY IN PREVIOUS LIFE-HISTORY

A *Individual pathology*
(a) traumatic experiences: surgical operations, serious illnesses, accidents, etc.;
(b) psychosomatic pathology.

93

B *Womanhood*
(a) gynaecological-obstetrical pathology;
(b) abnormality in sexual knowledge;
(c) negative incidents connected with feminine role;
(d) disturbances connected with feminine role: sexual problems, frigidity, etc.

C *Family background*
(a) traumatic events: death, accidents, deportation;
(b) pathology;
(c) interpersonal disturbances: misunderstandings, conflicts;
(d) disturbances in the structure of the family background: parents divorced, foster-parents, etc.

Note: categories (a), (b), (c) are scored separately for the following: mother, father, husband, other members of the family circle.

D *Social life*
(a) financial difficulties;
(b) difficulties of social and occupational adjustment.

II NEGATIVITY DURING PREGNANCY

A *General pathology*

B *Gynaecological-obstetrical pathology*

C *Psychosomatic symptoms specific to pregnancy*

D *Abnormal attitudes to motherhood*

E *Psychopathological symptoms*
(a) in relation to the woman herself: anxiety concerning childbirth, etc.;
(b) in relation to the child: fear of having an abnormal child, etc.;
(c) undefined: nightmares, etc.

F *Personality and behaviour disorders*
irritability, depression, etc.

G *Traumatic events and pathology in family circle, disturbances of interpersonal relations*

Note: these categories are scored separately for: mother, family of origin, husband, husband's family.

H *Social and economic difficulties*
problems connected with housing, work, etc.

DEFINITION OF ITEMS AND PRINCIPLES OF SCORING

I NEGATIVITY IN PREVIOUS LIFE-HISTORY

A *Individual pathology*

(a) Traumatic experiences:
surgical operations: serious operations or any, even minor, operations experienced as traumatic (an appendicectomy will always be scored, a tonsillectomy only when it appears to have been traumatic or regarded as important);

physical accidents: injuries, falls, etc.; a traumatic accident is scored even if it has involved no physical damage (for example, a fall from a bicycle in childhood, which has caused no bodily harm but has left distressful memories);

any important kind of pathology, hence all serious illnesses, which are, by definition, regarded as traumatic (diphtheria, tuberculosis, fits of depression, etc.).

Note: a traumatic experience associated with the subject's birth, when it involves definite pathology, is recorded under A(a) (e.g. neonatal anoxia, resuscitation).

(b) Psychosomatic pathology:
this category covers all forms of functional disorder, with a fairly low criterion for inclusion—

minor or chronic pathology: disorders of respiratory system (recurrent tonsillitis, etc.); bilious attacks, eczema, cystitis, enteritis, arterial hypertension, headaches, etc.;

mild neurotic symptoms: insomnia, irritability, depression, anxiety, palpitations, etc.

Note: abnormalities of development during childhood are also recorded under A(b) (e.g. late development, anorexia, enuresis).

B *Womanhood*

(a) Gynaecological-obstetrical pathology:
fibroma, cysts, metritis, metrorrhagia, vaginismus, etc.;
miscarriages;
disturbance of menstrual cycle: amenorrhoea, dysmenorrhoea;
presumed sterility (retroversion of the uterus, etc.).

Gynaecological pathology is recorded at a very low level; definite pathology is always circled (in particular, a miscarriage).

(b) Sexual and obstetrical information:
lack of information: not given information about first period or about sex, etc.;

negative or guilt-laden information about sex;

negative or traumatic information about pregnancy or childbirth: difficult or painful confinements experienced by someone close to subject (recorded at a particularly low level if the mother is concerned); this kind of information is always recorded in adulthood regardless of the period at which the incident took place; it may also be recorded under family pathology (mother or 'others').

(c) Negative incidents in the course of development of womanhood:
failures or traumatic emotional experiences in relation to role as a woman: breaking off of love affair, forced separation, emotional conflicts, etc.;

family or social problems connected with marriage (except financial difficulties);

miscarriages (already recorded under B(a)).

(d) Disturbances connected with feminine role:
parents wanted boy when subject was born;

rejection of feminine role: boys' games, narcissistic problems;

self-blame, rejection of womanhood, or refusal to assume womanhood fully, avoidance or fear of the other sex, menstrual trauma;

traumatic experience in first flirtation, traumatic experience in first intercourse (trivial report of painful first intercourse is not recorded if this does not appear to have had real negative significance);

frigidity, avoidance of sexual relations, negative valuation of sex.

C *Family background*

(a) Traumatic events:
death (always circled if it is of father or mother; if of other members of family, circled only when it has clearly been traumatic);

serious surgical operations undergone by a member of the family circle;

serious accident to one of family circle;

traumatic experiences due to outside events: connected with the war, displacement, deportation, etc.

Note: criterion for inclusion is higher than for individual traumatic experiences.

(b) Pathology:
as for A(b), but with a more exacting criterion for inclusion.

Note: only for gynaecological-obstetrical pathology of the mother is the criterion for inclusion low.

(c) Disturbances of interpersonal relations:
separation from parents in childhood, emotional rejection by parents (always circled);

conflicts or misunderstandings with member of family circle.

Note: particularly lenient criterion for inclusion of anything concerning the mother (failure of the mother to provide information on sexual matters is recorded under this heading);
headings (a), (b), and (c) require separate entries for mother, father, husband (from the period of adulthood), and for other members of the family circle.

(d) Disturbances in the structure of the family circle or in family attachments:
death or prolonged absence of one parent, parents separated, lived outside the family circle during childhood or adolescence;

bad family atmosphere, misunderstanding, quarrels between parents, etc.;

after marriage, couple not sufficiently independent of parents and parents-in-law; couple have difficulties in family relations: mixed marriage, one of partners previously divorced, living together without being married, etc.

D *Social life*

(a) Financial difficulties:
poverty, unemployment, difficulties over housing.

(b) Disturbances of social adjustment:
difficulties at school: failure, marked backwardness, interrupted education implying conflict or frustration;

difficulties at work: lack of occupational training felt acutely, unsatisfying job, occupational instability, interruption of work implying conflict or frustration;

disturbances of social relationships: difficulties in making contacts, social isolation, lack of self-confidence in social activities neurotic demanding attitudes.

97

II NEGATIVITY DURING PREGNANCY

A *General pathology*

all pathological manifestations, even psychosomatic, except psychosomatic symptoms specific to pregnancy (C).

Note: criterion for inclusion is lower than for the preceding periods; infectious diseases (e.g. rubella) which might affect the development of the pregnancy and the baby are always circled; other illnesses are circled when they are reacted to with anxiety (influenza, etc.).

B *Gynaecological-obstetrical pathology*

metrorrhagia, threatened abortion, uterine colic, leucorrhoea (important when its significance is exaggerated);

threat of premature delivery, extended pregnancy, abnormal presentation.

C *Specific psychosomatic symptoms*

symptoms considered: vomiting, nausea, lumbar pains, headaches, constipation, disturbed sleep, debility, excessive gaining of weight, breathlessness, tachycardia, dizziness;

symptoms are recorded globally: a plain cross is entered when at least two or three of these symptoms occur; a circled cross is entered when more than three symptoms occur, or when certain symptoms are particularly marked or their importance is exaggerated, or finally when they are accompanied by a high degree of debility (e.g. necessitating giving up work).

Note: some isolated symptoms may also be recorded (with plain cross or circled cross) when they have very great pathological significance: in particular, severe or persistent vomiting (hyperemesis).

D *Abnormal attitudes to motherhood*

failure to accept the child, fear of not knowing how to care for it;

sexual problems: rejection of or antipathy towards sexual activity (excluding fears for the baby); dyspareunia.

E *Psychopathological symptoms*

all forms of anxiety relating to pregnancy and childbirth are recorded here: acknowledged fears, fantasies, nightmares, etc.

anxieties relating to the woman herself: fear of childbirth (fear of dying or of suffering), narcissistic fears (relative to physical disfigurement);

anxieties relating to the child: fear of abnormality, fear of premature birth, etc.;

vague anxieties, anxiety dreams.

F *Personality and behaviour disorders*

irritability, touchiness, depressive tendencies (these last are recorded with a circled cross when they are fairly marked).

G *Family troubles*

traumatic experiences, pathology, and interpersonal disturbances, defined as in the first part of the grid, are all recorded here.

Note: separate entries are made for: mother, family of origin, husband, and husband's family.

H *Social and economic difficulties*

problems of accommodation created or aggravated by the coming of the baby; living with family or husband's family;

occupational problems created by the coming of the baby: enforced interruption of highly valued employment;

social problems raised by pregnancy before marriage.

SCORING OF CONFINEMENTS

The detailed review in Chapter 3 of the work done on, and the problems involved in, the assessment of confinements avoids the necessity for more than a brief explanation of the tool used in the present research. It should be noted first, however, that, because of the need for a standardized procedure, the scoring of confinements inevitably ignores a considerable range of data which might be of the greatest importance for a comprehensive and dynamic view of the experience of childbirth.

The system of scoring we adopted was simply intended to be more convenient, more detailed, and perhaps more 'accurate', than systems put forward hitherto.

In the first place, the main constituent of any quantitative assessment of confinement must surely be some index that takes account both of pain and of the nature of the behaviour exhibited. It has already been indicated that it is easier, quantitatively, to consider negative and objective factors. Since negative and positive aspects cannot be included in the same score, the pain and behaviour indices

99

were assigned by reference to an ideal norm rather than to interpretative standards. For pain, the ideal norm was complete analgesia; for behaviour, a completely neutral, inexpressive pattern. It will, of course, be realized that the fact that a woman conformed to such ideal norms would not necessarily imply a satisfactory confinement from a more comprehensive point of view. The pain-behaviour index as described below may be said, then, to reflect a certain negative quality of the confinement; it is, in short, the counterpart of the negativity index obtained from the grid presented above.

Second, the inadequacy of such an index for assessing confinements was partly offset by three factors:

(a) The use of a simply defined *obstetrical index*, which enabled differences between confinements *at the obstetrical level* to be taken into consideration.

(b) For more detailed investigation certain quantified factors were examined without any *a priori* implications of 'positive' or 'negative' significance. An account will be given later of such use of *indices* referring to the women's *activity, relation to others*, and *relation to the baby*.

(c) Finally a simple analysis applicable only to the prepared women indicated the extent to which the techniques taught during preparation were used, and how effective they were. (The other indices are, of course, essentially applicable to all parturient women.)

It did not seem possible to go further in refining an instrument which was intended, it must be remembered, as the counterpart of the negativity grid, even though it by no means records all the data available on the confinements.

DESCRIPTION OF THE CONFINEMENT GRID

The behaviour-pain indices

Essentially, the behaviour index (cf. Chapter 3) is as objective as possible: it takes account of every departure of behaviour from an ideal neutral standard. It thus includes all kinds of expressive manifestations such as screams, moans, gestures, grimaces, and verbalizations, without regard to their possible significance (as signs of pain or anxiety, or as expressive reactions characteristic of the woman).

In contrast, the pain index is frankly interpretative. It makes as much use of objective records as of obstetrical data (physical condition, length of labour, drugs), the subsequent account given by the woman, and knowledge of her defence mechanisms, her mode of expression, and her capacity for objectification.

For both pain and behaviour, a five-point scale was used, from category 1 (indicating complete analgesia on the one hand, and completely silent and neutral behaviour on the other) to category 5 (indicating the greatest intensity and lowest tolerance of pain, and the most clamorous and disorganized behaviour).

This double assessment was made on four distinct occasions, for the successive periods, respectively, of dilatation, transition, expulsion, and issue.

This division was empirically based, and is justified particularly by the correlations within each period (cf. Chapter 6). At the moment, it is sufficient to remark that, in view of the fact that a global index necessarily involves addition, it seemed best to treat dilatation and expulsion similarly in spite of their differences (in duration and in the nature of the problems of adjustment involved). The differentiation within each of these main phases (into dilatation and transition, expulsion and issue) meant that a more accurate picture could be obtained of the two brief but crucial stages during childbirth indicated by the terms transition and issue. The justification for this procedure will be found in the internal correlations between the partial indices, and their respective contributions to the global index.

This double entry, repeated four times for each confinement, provides:

(i) a global index, obtained by adding together all the entries, which indicates roughly the degree of negativity or unsatisfactoriness of the confinement;

(ii) a number of partial indices, obtained by adding columns (e.g. index of pain for the whole confinement) or rows (e.g. global index, including both pain and behaviour, for the expulsion period); comparison of the different indices yields interesting information on the various aspects of confinement and the relations between them; and these partial indices, as well as the global index, may be correlated with the global or partial indices obtained from the negativity grid.

Other indices

As has been stated, the inadequacy of this grid was corrected by certain procedures:

An *obstetrical index*, applied to each of the periods referred to above, yielded invaluable information in a very simple way. This index comprised three categories:

Category 1 implied that, in the period in question, there was no obstetrical problem, as testified by the form filled in by the obstetrician or midwife.

Category 3 implied that, in the period concerned, there was an obstetrical problem sufficiently serious to invalidate the global index. For example, arrested dilatation with oedema of the cervix and intravenous transfusion of posterior pituitary extract would make it hard to interpret the pain-behaviour index for the dilatation phase. Similarly, the use of forceps would imply that the index for the expulsion phase could not be used. This does not necessarily involve recourse to exclusively organic determinants which, by definition, would exclude the problem of the behaviour and the painful experience of the parturient woman, since psychological problems may underlie these obstetrical complications (a forceps delivery may be the result of psychological factors). It simply means that, at the level of the present research, the direct comparison of indices derived from such cases with indices for other parturient women is methodologically dubious.

Category 2 provided for the recording of common-place incidents (normal use of drugs, temporary slowing down of the process, preventive episiotomy, etc.), without any implication that comparison with other confinements would necessarily be affected.

Activity and the nature of relations with others and with the baby were assessed as follows. The schematic, fragmentary, and interpretative nature of these assessments will immediately be apparent.

Activity was assessed by assigning the woman to one of the three descriptive categories, active, neutral, and passive, without any implication that these formed a scale. This assessment did not depend directly on control or on the practice of technique. A woman might, for example, show poor control, yet be alert and participant; conversely, while practising the techniques, a woman might remain fundamentally passive. The assessment here interprets the global attitude of the woman throughout her confinement in so far as this attitude indicates a certain kind of 'alertness'.

Relation to others involves an assessment of a kind that it is particularly difficult to systematize. The woman's relation to those with whom she is in contact depends partly upon her general interpersonal relations, partly upon what she expects from those concerned and on the variable nature of such interpersonal relations, and partly upon the various counter-attitudes adopted towards the patient by midwives, nurses, and obstetrician. The dynamic way in which these various factors come together is an essentially individual matter. Two items were, however, selected for use *conjointly*, the significance of each depending upon the other:

the quality of the relationship as a whole (good, neutral, poor);
the intensity of the relationship (strong, average, weak).

In this way we obtained nine possible ratings, obviously of varying degrees of prominence and importance, as will be seen later.

Relation to the baby presents the same problem as does the previous dimension, and the same two items were retained:

the quality of the relationship (good, neutral or ambivalent, poor);
the intensity of the relationship (strong, average, weak).

Finally, for the detailed assessment of the *effects of preparation*, a three-point scale was used for breathing, relaxation, and bearing down, each treated separately. These assessments were made on two levels: in terms of the extent to which the techniques were used, and in terms of how effective they were (good results, average results, no effect).

ANALYSIS OF RESULTS

Each of the 116 case-histories retained for the final analysis (90 prepared and 26 unprepared women) was examined and recorded in terms of the two grids described above. Several methodological precautions were taken to ensure that the scores thus compiled would be as valid as possible:

The scoring was always effected a long time after the woman had been examined, and in series. Thus, all the entries in the negativity grid were made sequentially through the whole set of 116 case-histories, and then the same histories were gone over again to obtain the entries concerning confinement.

This scoring was always 'blind', the person who was recording being careful not to refer to the rest of the case-history; in particular, he avoided anything relating to the confinement when he was assessing negativity, and vice versa.

The material in each case-history was scored independently by two judges, who then compared their assessments. If these did not agree, the two judges proceeded to discuss their differences with a view to reaching an agreed decision (a method which is as a rule preferable to the easier solution of taking the mean of the two ratings proposed).

When all the entries were completed, 98 items of information, henceforth called 'variables', were isolated and examined for every woman, as follows:

15 general variables: age, years married, socio-economic level, sociocultural level, etc.;

50 negativity variables, ranging from the partial indices for areas and periods (more or less specific) to the global indices representing negativity in the personal history (Total I), negativity during pregnancy (Total II), and overall or general negativity (Totals I + II);

33 variables relating to the confinement, again ranging from the more specific to the more global.

The level of measurement used in establishing these variables varies considerably. In some cases, the variables are genuine quasi-continuous variables (such as the global index of negativity, which shows a range of from 8 to 40, with many intermediate values). In other cases, only three- or four-point scales are involved (e.g. with respect to the use of PPM techniques). This second category would include cases where an underlying, theoretically continuously distributed, variable had been arbitrarily divided into two, three, or more classes for

104

reasons of convenience (e.g. the six sociocultural levels). Finally, in some cases, only the simplest possible form of measurement was used: the division into two mutually exclusive classes (e.g. Jewish or non-Jewish).

In all these cases, the information concerning the woman was indicated by a number (e.g. global negativity index = 27; use of breathing techniques = 0 (good); sociocultural level = 1 (low); non-Jewish = 0, Jewish = 1).

These 98 variables were recorded on punched cards for each of the 116 women. Two statistical analyses were then processed by computer, one for the prepared women and one for the unprepared women. The result of these analyses, in respect of each group, was to provide:

(a) mean and standard deviation for each of the 98 variables;

(b) all the possible correlations among these 98 variables, taken in pairs, i.e. 4,753 correlations (product-moment coefficients). The coefficient of correlation used was Bravais-Pearson's r. This measure is particularly appropriate for variables with a number of classes, such as the global index of negativity or the global confinement score, but there is no reason why it should not be applied where only a small number of classes are involved, even two.

For some minor analyses (see especially Chapter 8), it was necessary to work with subgroups of women selected from the total population according to certain criteria. This analysis, carried out by more 'everyday' methods, sometimes used other coefficients of correlation (especially Spearman's rank-difference coefficient ρ, and the tetrachoric correlation r). Finally, the statistical significance of the differences in means and standard deviations between groups was estimated in general either by Student's t or by Fisher's χ^2.

The results obtained will be examined and discussed in the next three chapters.

SUMMARY

Two new instruments were developed for the purposes of the present research, the negativity grid and the confinement scoring grid.

The negativity grid summarizes, classifies, and quantifies the data derived from the interviews, but deals, as its name indicates, only with negative or unfavourable items: traumatic experiences and illness of various kinds, unfavourable incidents and circumstances, etc., which,

105

broadly speaking, might be regarded as constituting a burden of liabilities, the effect of which upon pregnancy and childbirth can be investigated.

The negativity grid thus provides a systematic inventory of negative items and enables these to be quantified. All these items, however, do not receive equal weight. An attempt was made to give special importance to those items that appeared likely, on theoretical grounds, to have the most direct effects upon pregnancy and childbirth. This was done in two ways, by increasing the number of entries to be made in the area concerned, and by making more lenient the criteria by which items were judged of sufficient importance to be included. In this way, for example, were recorded the negative items relating to the problems of womanhood.

The negativity grid was developed in two stages. A preliminary version was used with 60 case-histories, and the results obtained enabled a critical analysis of the instrument to be made, on the basis of which it was modified. The second and final form, used in the main research, enabled recording to be done more rapidly, and on a more rational and better integrated basis.

The instrument comprised two parts. The first part recorded negativity in the personal history of the subject, in three separate periods (childhood, adolescence, and adulthood); the second part recorded negativity during pregnancy, with the earlier and later stages of pregnancy distinguished. Several areas of interest were distinguished within each of the main parts: individual pathology, womanhood, family background, and social life, for negativity in the personal history; general pathology, gynaecological-obstetrical pathology, symptoms specific to pregnancy, abnormalities in maternal attitude, psychopathological symptoms specific to pregnancy (anxieties), personality disorders, family background, and social life, for negativity during pregnancy.

In this way there was obtained for each woman a series of partial scores (one for each area in each period) which could be added both by areas and by periods. It was also possible to get a score for each of the two main parts (negativity in personal history and negativity during pregnancy), and a total score was obtained by adding the scores for these two parts (the global negativity score).

In a similar way a second grid was constructed, aimed at summarizing, classifying, and quantifying the observations relating to confinement. At four stages during the confinement (dilatation, transition, expulsion, issue) two aspects were assessed quantitatively on an appropriate scale: the quality of behavioural control and, in a more interpretative way, the pain experienced. Here again, various summations were possible: to obtain a global score (pain *plus* behavioural control) for a given period (e.g. during dilatation), or to obtain an assessment of the confinement as a whole (whether in terms of pain or behaviour, or of both together).

Several aspects which it was thought preferable to note separately were excluded from this global index because it seemed undesirable and technically difficult to try to combine them additively with the aspects mentioned above to give a single score. This was the case with the activity shown by the woman during labour, her relations with other people in the labour ward, and her first relationship to the baby, which were therefore assessed separately. Similarly, in the case of prepared women, the use of PPM techniques (breathing, relaxation, and bearing down) was recorded separately. Finally, for all cases, the information was completed by a statement of the obstetrical features of the confinement, summarized in an 'obstetrical index'.

Two main types of statistical treatment were applied to these data: an analysis of the distributions of the different variables was useful particularly for comparing the prepared and unprepared women; and a study of the correlations between variables was valuable both for clarifying the psychometric structure of the instruments themselves and for investigating the relationships between negativity and childbirth.

CHAPTER 6

The Confinements

Before embarking upon the study of the relations between negativity and confinement, which is the main concern of our research, it will be useful to examine the confinements themselves, as they appear in the data collected.

We have attempted to express, by means of indices as closely standardized and as accurately quantified as possible, certain characteristics of the confinements observed in our sample population. Our first task is to review the results obtained. It must, of course, be remembered that these results are largely dependent upon the criteria used during the observation, and later during the assessment, of the confinements. The significance of the results obtained must therefore be discussed in the light of the methodological assumptions made and the techniques employed in the research, as expounded in Chapter 3.

The present chapter reports the results in terms of the various dimensions derived from the grid, as explained in Chapter 5. One of the main aspects of our exposition and discussion will be the comparison of the prepared and the unprepared women. We shall consider, in the following order:

(a) the global confinement index and its components, pain and behavioural control, on the one hand, and the partial indices relevant to the different periods, on the other;

(b) the relations between the global index and certain obstetrical features of the confinements;

(c) the more qualitative aspects of childbirth: activity, relation to other people and to the baby, and their relations with the global index;

(d) the use of PPM techniques and their effectiveness in prepared women.

THE GLOBAL CONFINEMENT INDEX AND ITS COMPONENTS

We shall examine, first, the results obtained for the group of 90 women prepared by the PPM, and only after the main features of these findings have been established shall we proceed to compare the prepared and unprepared women.

It will be remembered that the global index is obtained by adding eight partial scores, each of which may vary from 1 to 5 (pain scores and behaviour scores for each of four distinct stages of the confinement). The possible range of this index is therefore from 8 to 40, a score of 8 representing a 'perfect' confinement in terms of the criteria adopted. It is, of course, extremely unlikely that one would actually come across a score of 8, and this represents, in effect, an ideal standard of reference.

DISTRIBUTION OF THE GLOBAL INDEX

Figure 1 gives the distribution of the global scores for the 90 women prepared by the PPM. This distribution shows a wide scatter, the scores spreading over the greater part of the possible range. The global index therefore discriminates adequately, and effectively reflects the differences observable between the women.

Figure 1   Distribution of global confinement scores for 90 prepared women

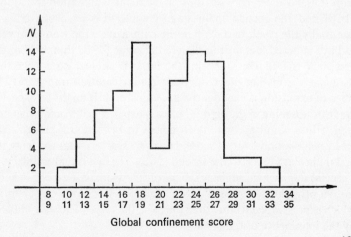

Global confinement score

The mean was 21·15, slightly lower than the mid-point of the possible range. Thus the average confinement was a little better than that indicated by the mid-point of 24·00. There are, however, relatively few scores near the mean, and, on either side, two subgroups emerge which are clearly distinguishable in respect of quality of confinement as assessed by our method. It may be observed in passing that the observed distribution agrees quite well with immediate clinical intuition. The clinicians who scored the observations made of the confinements had in fact commented, before any overall statistical analysis was undertaken, that confinements which had been judged 'good' by a global estimate at the time of observation corresponded in general to scores of less than 21 or 22, while the 'poor' confinements corresponded to higher scores.

COMPONENTS OF THE GLOBAL INDEX

For a better understanding of the characteristics of the distribution of the global scores, it is useful to analyse the partial scores making up the global index and see how they combine.

Table 5 enables us to compare the pain scores and the behavioural control scores, and also to compare the scores for the different stages of the confinement. It will be seen that, for the confinement as a whole (all stages combined), the 90 women obtain very similar average scores for both pain (10·60) and control (10·67). The average global score falls, however, between the first main stage (dilatation-transition, 11·50) and the second main stage (expulsion-issue, 9·65). This is essentially the result of a drop in the pain score – the women appear to have suffered less during the second stage (4·60) than during the first stage (6·00). This confirms the familiar clinical experience that the most 'distressing' stage of childbirth is dilatation-transition. The stage of expulsion is experienced as less painful. It might be expected that this lessening in the amount of pain experienced would be associated with a simultaneous improvement in behavioural control; the mean behavioural control score, however, scarcely changes from the first main stage (5·44) to the second (5·12). The fact is that expulsion is a crucial stage which subjects the parturient woman to stress; in some cases it provokes a degree of disorganization of activity and of control which expresses, even more than the pain, the surge of anxiety induced by the imminence of the birth.

110

TABLE 5 MEANS AND STANDARD DEVIATIONS OF CONFINEMENT
SCORES FOR PREPARED AND UNPREPARED GROUPS

			Stages 1 Dila-tation	2 Trans-ition	3 Expul-sion	4 Issue	*Stages combined* 1 + 2	3 + 4	Total
Pain	PPM	*m*	2·90	3·10	2·22	2·40	6·0	4·60	10·60
		σ	0·86	0·74	0·76	0·95	1·46	1·83	2·3
	U	*m*	(3·42)	(3·42)	(2·35)	(2·50)	(6·85)	(4·85)	(11·69)
		σ	(0·63)	(0·84)	(0·73)	(0·83)	(1·35)	(1·43)	(2·20)
Behaviour	PPM	*m*	2·50	2·94	2·63	2·49	5·44	5·12	10·67
		σ	1·17	1·08	1·03	1·11	2·06	1·98	3·6
	U	*m*	(3·35)	(3·46)	(2·92)	(2·73)	(6·81)	(5·65)	(12·46)
		σ	(1·07)	(1·05)	(1·03)	(1·06)	(1·98)	(1·90)	(3·30)
Total	PPM	*m*	5·41	6·09	4·87	4·79	11·50	9·65	21·15
		σ	1·87	1·54	1·61	1·80	3·15	3·12	5·26
	U	*m*	(6·77)	(6·85)	(5·27)	(5·19)	(13·65)	(10·12)	(24·15)
		σ	(1·50)	(1·63)	(1·61)	(1·80)	(2·92)	(2·91)	(4·92)

Note : In this and other tables, figures relating to the unprepared group (U) are given in parentheses.

Table 5 also indicates that the scatter of scores is greater for be-havioural control than for pain, i.e. that there are more differences between women with respect to degree of control manifested than with respect to amount of pain felt. It may well be that the more objective nature of the control score enables more effective use to be made of the five-point scale and a greater degree of differentiation to be achieved, whereas the more subjective nature of the pain score means that the rater more frequently uses the centre category, 3, to reflect his uncertainty, and a reduced scatter follows. It is very difficult here to decide what is an artefact of the scoring system and what reflects the true nature of the observed facts.

INTERRELATIONS BETWEEN PARTIAL SCORES AND CONSTITUTION OF THE TOTAL SCORE

An examination of the means cannot in itself show the importance of the partial scores as constituents of the global score. This requires a correlational study which takes account both of the correlations between the partial scores themselves, and of the correlations of each of the partial scores with the global score.

If the pain and behaviour scores are examined separately, they appear to contribute approximately equally to the global score for the whole confinement (correlations of 0·86 and 0·90 respectively with the global score); in other words, the global score is not affected more by one of these aspects than by the other. Despite the fact that both the pain score and the behavioural control score contribute equally and substantially to the total score, they each yield somewhat different information, as is indicated by their intercorrelation (0·62) which, though appreciable, leaves each measure with a substantial amount of specific variance, as indeed was the intention. The point of distinguishing between the two measures will be clarified by an analysis of results as related to the different stages.

As far as these stages are concerned, it is found that the first stage (dilatation-transition) contributes as much to the total score as does the second stage (expulsion-issue): the correlations calculated separately between the partial totals for each of these two stages (including both pain and behavioural control) and the global total are the same (0·84).

But if one looks at the differences between the pain and the control scores, on the one hand, in conjunction with the differences between stages, on the other, indications of interesting patterns over time appear. Examination of the correlations reveals that partial scores for control, for successive periods, remain relatively similar for the same woman: a woman who shows good control during dilatation and transition has a good chance of also showing good control during expulsion and issue (correlation between control scores for the two stages, 0·50). On the other hand, the pain experienced during dilatation-

112

transition is not an effective predictor of the pain that will be experienced during expulsion and issue (correlation, 0·17). This last finding emphasizes the advantage of assessing separately the two stages of childbirth. In most of the previous work referred to in Chapter 3, the authors have not gone beyond a single global assessment for the whole confinement. The present research gives clear indication of *temporal factors*, which may well be of considerable importance for the understanding of individual confinements. These temporal factors appear to be connected mainly with pain and its variations during confinement. We have seen that the average pain score is less in the expulsion stage than in the dilatation-transition stage, and it is clear that, for any given woman, pain tends to vary considerably between stages according to patterns of development over time of an individual nature.

Finally, the difference between the pain score and the behaviour score was calculated for every woman for each stage. This was expressed as pain score *minus* behaviour score. Thus a positive difference indicated that the woman concerned had a higher score for pain than for behaviour, and that the pain she appeared to experience was greater than the disorganization of behaviour she showed. Conversely, a negative difference indicated that the disorganization of behaviour the woman showed was greater than the pain she apparently felt. The distribution of differences was worked out for each stage of confinement, and the means and standard deviations were calculated. An examination of these means confirms the results referred to above: the mean of the differences between the pain and behaviour scores reflects the differences observed between the means of the two variables, separately calculated (*Table 5*). The scatter of the difference remains roughly constant for all four stages. The most interesting thing about it is probably that, at every stage, it is sufficiently great to suggest that the difference between the two scores reflects an individual variable which characterizes the style of confinement.

Qualitatively, three groups of women may be distinguished: women with very effective control, whose behaviour is not an adequate indication of the pain they feel; women who spontaneously express the pain they feel without however amplifying it in their behavioural manifestations; and women with especially poor control, who behave theatrically and whose behaviour tends to give the impression that they are experiencing more pain than is in fact the case. These difference scores may be regarded as reflecting the *level of control*, and

113

may be correlated with the confinement indices themselves. Correlations were in fact calculated between the total scores (pain plus behaviour) for each of the two main stages of confinement (dilatation-transition and expulsion-issue) and the difference scores (pain minus behaviour) for the corresponding stages. The coefficients were 0·39 for the first stage and 0·38 for the second stage. *The women with better control therefore appear to have the better overall confinements.* Should we conclude from this that good control favours a good confinement, or that good control is itself more likely to be the result of an easy confinement? Here, as generally, the existence of a correlation does not in itself enable us to decide the direction of causality, and interpretation in either sense is possible. The most plausible interpretation, however, would appear to be that women prepared by the PPM are specifically provided with the means of controlling their manifestations of pain, are better able to do so in so far as they are not too overwhelmed by pain, and consequently have a relatively easy confinement.

Thus far, we have been concerned only with the results for the women prepared by the PPM. It was hoped that in this way the exposition would be simplified and the general pattern of the results more easily followed. Our next step is to compare the results for the prepared women with those for the control group represented by the unprepared women.

In *Table 5*, the means of the confinement scores (both global and partial) for the unprepared women are given in parentheses below the means for the prepared group. As might be expected, the global confinement score is higher for the unprepared women, indicating that they have, on average, less satisfactory confinements. *Figure 2*, which shows the distribution of the global scores for both groups, illustrates the same difference even more clearly. In particular, nearly half of the prepared women (44 per cent) have a score of less than 20, i.e. fall within the category of 'good' confinements, whereas this is the case for only a small proportion of the unprepared women (11 per cent). *Table 5* further shows that the poorer quality of confinement for unprepared women is reflected in all the partial scores. It is, however, more marked in respect of the behavioural control scores than in respect of the pain scores. It is also more marked during the first stage than during the second. It was, of course, only to be expected that prepared women would have better confinements in comparison with

114

unprepared women. Considered as a whole, the present results simply confirm what numerous other studies had already established, namely, the effectiveness of preparation.

It is more interesting to consider for which aspects of confinement and for which stages this beneficial effect is most apparent. The fact that it is more marked in respect of behavioural control than of pain is also

Figure 2   Comparison of global confinement scores for 90 prepared women and 26 unprepared women

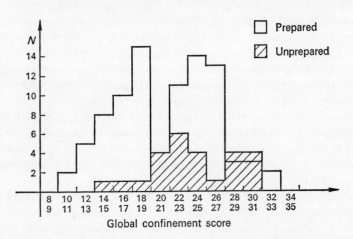

in keeping with previous findings. Preparation essentially furnishes a model of behaviour to which the women try to adhere. By conforming to the behavioural norms learned in the course of preparation the women meet the expectations of the personnel of the labour ward, in so far as the obstetricians and midwives themselves adhere to the same norms. Thus success depends both upon the satisfactory use of the techniques taught and upon a good adjustment to the personnel of the labour ward, effected through the relationships established with the hospital staff. According to the PPM, analgesia is achieved as a result of preparation partly because it facilitates the active and conscious use of special techniques (and more generally of learned models of behaviour) and partly because it provides the opportunity for harmonious integration within a network of interpersonal relations, which brings the woman the emotional support she needs.

It is therefore scarcely surprising that analgesia, in so far as it is an indirect consequence of more effective behaviour and of adjustment to the expectations of the labour ward, should be less clearly manifest than the behavioural adjustment itself. The fact that it is noticeable at all is sufficient to provide at least partial confirmation for the preliminary hypotheses of the PPM.

It is also of interest to find that the improvement brought about by the PPM is more pronounced during the dilatation-transition stage than during the expulsion-issue stage.

To summarize, the difference between prepared and unprepared women is particularly marked during the dilatation-transition stage and, as was shown above, in respect of behavioural control. It is worth underlining this somewhat paradoxical fact that the PPM is most liable to influence behavioural control during the dilatation-transition stage when this same period is the most painful stage of childbirth. This may, however, become comprehensible if it is assumed that, while the dilatation-transition stage is undoubtedly the most painful, more anxiety is involved in the expulsion-issue stage. In this case, it would be easier for preparation to control manifestations of pain than to control the signs of disorganization of behaviour which accompany a powerful upsurge of anxiety.

Valuable support for these findings is given by a consideration of the differences between the pain scores and the behaviour scores of the unprepared women, and of the correlations between these differences and the confinement scores for the different stages. If we compare the difference scores of the unprepared women with those of the prepared women, the means of the unprepared women are found to be systematically displaced in the negative direction for all four stages. This indicates that the unprepared women on average show poorer control than do the prepared women. This finding is a natural consequence of the results already considered above, which indicated that the prepared women were superior especially in behavioural control. Moreover, the scatter of difference scores is the same for both groups of women and in both broups is the same for the different stages. The implication would appear to be that preparation simply raises the average level of control, without reducing the range of individual differences. It does not seem to have very much effect upon personal style in so far as this depends upon factors of personality.

116

An interesting difference appears between the two groups, however, when we consider the correlations between level of control and confinement score. Whereas the correlations between difference scores (pain minus control) and total confinement scores (pain plus control) are very similar in prepared and unprepared women for the dilatation-transition stage (0·39 for prepared and 0·45 for unprepared), the correlation is much higher for the unprepared women during the expulsion-issue stage (0·38 for prepared and 0·77 for unprepared). In the latter stage, therefore, the level of control is closely related to the overall quality of the confinement for unprepared women. It is interesting to consider several possible interpretations of this finding. It might at first appear that the unprepared women tend to show better control during this stage, the more easily their confinement is proceeding. In that case, however, one would have to explain why preparation has the effect of weakening this relationship, when it has no effect upon the relationship observed for the first stage. Again, according to this hypothesis, preparation should have a particularly beneficial effect on behaviour during the expulsion-issue stage; and, as we have seen, it is in fact during the dilatation-transition stage that this beneficial effect is most noticeable. This contradiction therefore casts doubt upon the first of these possible explanations. It is perhaps simpler to assume that in unprepared women a level of control which rises spontaneously during the expulsion-issue stage is particularly favourable to a good confinement at this period. In unprepared women, indeed, a controlled attitude may well be more closely connected with more fundamental personality patterns, and may reflect well-adjusted defence mechanisms which allow them to offset the anxiety associated with the birth; whereas in prepared women, who have learned for the occasion, and therefore more superficially, to adopt controlled behaviour, this increase in anxiety is more likely merely to be camouflaged in behaviour. For prepared women, good apparent control would then be less likely to be associated with a good confinement in this particularly anxiety-laden stage.

On the whole, our results suggest that the benefits derived from the PPM, although undeniable, nevertheless remain at a relatively superficial level and are accompanied only to a limited extent by the reduction of anxiety that one might expect to find. At the most anxious moments during confinement, the women's reactions are essentially determined by their individual psychological structure, and preparation has little effect. Confirmation of this hypothesis will be sought in a later study of the correlations between negativity and quality of confinement at the different stages.

A correlational analysis was also made of the relative contributions of the partial scores to the global confinement score for the unprepared women. It is worth noting that, even although the mean confinement scores for the two groups of women are different, especially in the case of some of the constituent sub-scores, the correlations between partial scores and total score are almost identical in the two groups. This agreement in the two sets of results is of interest because it emphasizes the soundness of the instrument of assessment, which retains its internal structure (reflected in the correlations between partial scores and total score) even when it is applied to different groups, and enables clear differences in the nature of the data to be established.

INCIDENCE OF OBSTETRICAL FACTORS

The success of a confinement cannot be regarded exclusively from a psychological point of view, independently of the incidence of certain obstetrical factors. It is clinically clear that a confinement that is obstetrically difficult cannot be the same kind of psychological experience as one that is entirely 'normal'. For this reason, several obstetrical variables were taken into consideration in the present research.

OBSTETRICAL DATA USED

It will be remembered that the confinement grid contained a separate category for obstetrical incidents which might affect the course of the confinement. For each of the four stages distinguished, a three-point obstetrical scale was used:

a value of 3 was assigned when any incident of a clearly pathological nature occurred during the course of the confinement, which necessitated either medication or more than trivial intervention;

a value of 2 was assigned when there were insignificant incidents which were neither serious nor urgent;

a value of 1 was assigned when the confinement, at the stage in question, proceeded normally without requiring any form of medical intervention.

A few examples will illustrate the use of these criteria. An extremely long dilatation, because of rigidity of the cervix, for example, needing heavy medication, would be given a value of 3; so would an issue requiring forceps for any reason whatever. A rather long dilatation requiring mild medication, or an episiotomy at the moment of issue, or a natural tear, would be given a value of 2.

It should be emphasized that any obstetrical incidents serious enough to differentiate the confinements involved from others with regard to the probable effect of genuinely psychological factors, or to the nature of the subjective experience, were assigned a value of 3. The assigning of this value at any point during the confinement meant that the particular case was excluded from the experimental sample. All women who had had a forceps delivery were therefore excluded from the data on which the present analyses are based.

By comparison, the values 1 and 2 are not very different. The grounds on which one or the other value was decided upon were often of a situational nature (for example, the general features of the labour ward or the attitude of the midwives), since these aspects play an important part in decisions to use drugs or to perform an episiotomy, etc. A value of 2, therefore, was never given in a case where there were real pathological features, but only to indicate a kind of 'obstetrical inconvenience'.

These ratings were made separately for each stage and then added to provide a global obstetrical index, varying from 4 to 8 (a count of 1 or 2 for each of the four stages), since all cases receiving a value of 3 were eliminated.

The most frequently occurring score for this global obstetrical index is not 4, which would correspond to a complete absence of obstetrical incidents. Much more frequently, there are one or two incidents assigned a value of 2, with the result that the most frequent scores for the global index are 5 and 6. The means are 5·7 for the unprepared group and 5·2 for the prepared group. It is interesting to observe that such closely similar means are obtained for both groups. This no doubt reflects the relative lack of discrimination between the values 1 and 2 according to the definition of the two categories, since values of 3, which were taken as grounds for eliminating the case from the analysis, occur significantly more frequently in the unprepared women among whom there is, in particular, a relatively large number of forceps deliveries.

In addition to this obstetrical index, which is included in the main confinement grid presented in Chapter 5, a certain amount of other information was available, which was used in the overall statistical analysis:

(i) the duration of the confinement (labour was taken as beginning at two fingers dilatation and total duration was then up to and including issue; short confinements were considered to be those not exceeding ten hours);
(ii) the degree of medication (two groups were distinguished here, the first consisting of women having little or no medication, the second consisting of women having frequent or relatively heavy medication; a transfusion was always included in the second group);
(iii) weight of the baby at birth;
(iv) whether or not the confinement was at term.

These obstetrical data are clearly not mutually independent, but they are not too closely related, as *Table 6* indicates. Two correlations in particular stand out, that between length of labour and obstetrical

TABLE 6   INTERCORRELATIONS BETWEEN VARIOUS
OBSTETRICAL DATA

		Obstetrical index	*Duration*	*Medication*	*Baby's weight*
Duration	PPM U	+·24 (+·42)			
Medication	PPM U	+·21 (+·53)	+·36 (+·34)		
Baby's weight	PPM U	+·18 (+·12)	−·07 (+·28)	+·20 (−·06)	
Whether at term	PPM U	−·04 (+·05)	−·07 (+·27)	−·06 (−·19)	−·18 (+·04)

TABLE 7   CORRELATIONS BETWEEN DURATION OF
CONFINEMENT AND CONFINEMENT SCORES

| | | *Stages* | | | | *Stages combined* | | |
		1 *Dila-* *tation*	*2* *Trans-* *ition*	*3* *Expul-* *sion*	*4* *Issue*	*1+2*	*3+4*	*Total*
Pain	PPM	+·32	+·28	−·05	+·07	+·33	−·04	+·22
	U	(+·34)	(+·04)	(+·08)	(+·14)	(+·18)	(+·13)	(+·20)
Control	PPM	+·26	+·19	−·06	−·14	+·24	−·11	+·06
	U	(+·41)	(+·19)	(−·16)	(+·11)	(+·32)	(−·02)	(+·18)
Total	PPM	+·31	+·24	−·04	−·06	+·30	−·05	+·15
	U	(+·43)	(+·13)	(−·11)	(+·16)	(+·30)	(+·21)	(+·21)

index, and that between degree of medication and obstetrical index. These correlations show that the obstetrical inconvenience indicated by the index is related to both length of labour and degree of medication. This is scarcely surprising, since both of these were included in the criteria on the basis of which the obstetrical index was arrived at.

As far as the relations between the obstetrical variables and the confinement scores are concerned, the clearest findings involve the effects of the duration of labour. *Table 7* gives the correlations between the total duration of the confinement and the confinement scores (for pain and behavioural control, at the different stages). There is practically no relationship between the total duration of confinement and the global score. If, however, we examine the partial scores, there is a sizable correlation between total duration and the scores for the dilatation stage, which is higher for unprepared women (0·43) than for prepared women (0·31). For the former, duration has more effect upon behavioural control than upon pain, whereas for the latter, the reverse is the case, duration having greater influence upon the experience of pain. The observed correlation diminishes during transition and disappears altogether during expulsion-issue.

These results support fairly well those analysed earlier. Prepared women are able to offset the behavioural manifestations of pain or anxiety during dilatation, without deriving corresponding benefits in relation to suffering. The trying nature of a long labour therefore finds expression for them in the form of pain experienced rather than in the form of disorganization of behaviour. Unprepared women not only are affected by the accumulation of pain which prolonged dilatation tends to produce, but also experience more acutely its disorganizing effect upon behaviour; and it may well be that for them the manifestations of anxiety actually increase their expression of pain.

It must be remembered that, in interpreting the course of these correlations according to stages, we have taken account only of the total duration of the confinement and not of the relative durations of each of the stages involved; but it is clear that the total duration must depend largely on the duration of dilatation, so that it is not surprising that its effects are greatest during this stage.

The other obstetrical factors considered – the weight of the baby, the fact that the confinement has or has not occurred at term, the degree of medication – do not show any clear relationship with the confinement scores. This does not, of course, imply that these factors are of no consequence for the woman's experience of childbirth. Such a conclusion not only would offend clinical experience, but would be quite unjustified. First of all, it should be remembered that the categories used to provide the data for the calculation of the correlations are fairly coarse. They were, as such, intended only to provide a few reference points and not to enable an exhaustive analysis of these factors to be made. Moreover, a zero correlation is always difficult to interpret, since it can quite well mask real but complex relationships. For example, as a result of the intrusion of other variables, there might exist between two correlated variables a positive relationship for some women and a negative relationship for others, with the result that, for both these groups together, the correlation would be zero or negligible. As far as the relation between medication and confinement scores is concerned, the causal network is so complex that it is not surprising if no statistical relationship is evident. Medication is used most frequently in cases in which labour promises to be or is difficult. It should therefore be associated with higher pain scores and higher behavioural control scores. On the other hand, however, medication tends to reduce pain and to normalize the progress of the confinement, and would therefore offset the relationship posited.

STUDY OF THE QUALITATIVE ASPECTS OF CHILDBIRTH

The global index of the success of a confinement which we have considered in the preceding paragraphs is essentially no more than a quantitative assessment of pain and behavioural control. It should be remembered that these two aspects were selected because they seemed particularly suited to quantification and because they occupied a special position with respect to preparation by the PPM, the study of which is a main concern of the present investigation. The global index used appears to reflect reasonably well the success of the confinement, from this point of view. Our results, in that they indicate, as has been shown above, a marked difference between women prepared by the PPM and unprepared women, confirm that this is so.

In the preceding chapters, however, it has been emphasized that a complete description of a confinement from a psychological point of view should take account of certain other aspects, which will now be considered.

In the confinement grid, there are included three-point scales for each of three aspects of confinement of special importance for a psychological interpretation – activity, relations with staff, and relation to the baby. These variables have already been introduced and discussed in previous chapters, both with regard to their theoretical significance and with regard to the operational definitions given to them in our system of observation and classification. We now turn to the results obtained concerning each of these three aspects.

ACTIVITY

The mean on the three-point activity scale for the 90 women prepared by the PPM is 1·82, close to the value of 2 which represents the theoretical mean. For the 26 unprepared women, the mean is 1·62, not much different from the mean for the prepared women. This finding may

123

seem surprising if it is remembered that the notion of activity is one of the key notions of the PPM, according to which preparation should tend to make the women more active. But it must be emphasized that the definition of activity adopted in the present research is somewhat different from that propounded by the practitioners of the PPM. In particular, our definition gives much less weight, for the purpose of assessment, to activity involving the practice of PPM techniques. The

TABLE 8   CORRELATIONS BETWEEN ACTIVITY AND
CONFINEMENT SCORES

| | | Stages | | | | Stages combined | | |
		1 Dila- tation	2 Trans- ition	3 Expul- sion	4 Issue	1 + 2	3 + 4	Total
Pain	PPM	+·24	+·31	+·21	+·17	+·31	+·29	+·34
	U	(−·07)	(−·05)	(+·59)	(+·29)	(−·06)	(+·49)	(+·28)
Control	PPM	+·45	+·49	+·54	+·40	+·51	+·50	+·62
	U	(+·26)	(+·15)	(+·60)	(+·59)	(+·22)	(+·65)	(+·51)
Total	PPM	+·39	+·46	+·44	+·31	+·46	+·41	+·52
	U	(+·16)	(+·04)	(+·65)	(+·46)	(+·12)	(+·63)	(+·47)

extent to which these techniques are used and their effectiveness are handled separately. Here, we are concerned with the attempt to assess activity in a rather interpretative and global way, in which the assessment more or less corresponds to an estimate of the participation of the woman in the progress of her confinement and thus reflects an aspect of her involvement in the situation. Interpreted in this way, activity constitutes a very general individual variable with something of the sense in which it is used in characterology (as by Le Senne, for example). It may therefore be applied in the same kind of way to unprepared and prepared women. It is, however, interesting to note

124

that, in fact, the measure of activity does not differentiate between the two groups of women, although this finding may be a little misleading, since the sample of unprepared women is somewhat 'selected' in one relevant respect by the elimination of all cases of forceps delivery, which are more frequent among the unprepared than among the prepared women, and tend to occur among the least active women.

Clear relationships emerge between activity ratings and confinement scores, as is indicated in *Table 8*. The correlation between global confinement score and activity is reasonably high (prepared women, 0·52; unprepared women, 0·47), and it is, in fact, the behavioural control score that is most closely related to activity (prepared women, 0·62; unprepared women, 0·51). This association is obvious, in the sense in which activity is used here. We shall see later that there are also clear relationships between activity and the use of PPM techniques (breathing, relaxation, and bearing down), and we shall return to the question of the relations between activity and the other aspects of confinement. At the moment, we simply wish to underline that activity represents an important confinement variable both for unprepared women and for women prepared by the PPM, and that its correlations with other aspects of confinement are similar in both groups.

RELATIONS WITH STAFF

Under this heading we are concerned with the emerging pattern of interaction between the woman and the hospital and medical staff. This relationship depends upon a large number of both objective and subjective factors. The subjective factors are those relating to the personality of the parturient woman, in so far as this determines the demands that she makes upon the hospital and its staff, and her reactions to them. The personality of the midwife, in return, influences the nature of the interpersonal relations thus established. These develop, however, against a background of objective conditions, and will vary according to the time of day, the extent to which the labour ward is overcrowded, and so on.

The assessment that we made attempted to take account of the totality of interpersonal phenomena, including both subjective and objective aspects without distinguishing between them. To reflect this complex reality as faithfully as possible, a two-dimensional classification was adopted to take account of the quality and of the intensity of the relationship established. Each dimension was rated on a three-point scale as follows:

quality: positive (1); ambivalent (2); negative (3);
intensity: strong (1); average (2); weak (3).

These two dimensions taken together thus provided nine categories.

Table 9 shows how the women were divided among these nine categories. It is particularly interesting to examine this table from the point of view of comparing the percentages for the prepared and unprepared women. The prepared women, on the whole, more often have a positive relationship than do the unprepared (44 per cent against 27 per cent), and less often a negative relationship (9 per cent against 30·5 per cent), whereas an ambivalent relationship is about equally

TABLE 9 DISTRIBUTION OF PREPARED AND UNPREPARED
WOMEN WITH RESPECT TO INTENSITY AND QUALITY OF
RELATIONS WITH STAFF

Quality		Strong	Intensity Average	Weak	Total
		%	%	%	%
Positive	PPM	16	23	5	44
	U	(7·5)	(7·5)	(12)	(27)
Ambivalent	PPM	29	11	7	47
	U	(31)	(7·5)	(4)	(42.5)
Negative	PPM	4	5	0	9
	U	(19)	(7·5)	(4)	(30·5)
Total	PPM	49	39	12	
	U	(57·5)	(22·5)	(20)	

frequent in both groups. The two groups are less clearly differentiated with respect to the intensity of the relationship, though an average intensity of relationship is observed more frequently, and a strong or weak relationship less frequently, among the prepared women than among the unprepared.

It can be seen, from a combination of these two dimensions, that among the prepared women the categories representing a positive relationship of strong or average intensity have a relatively large number of entries, whereas the category representing a negative relationship of strong intensity has a relatively small number of entries. There is a clear group difference in this respect.

Among the unprepared women, the relationship therefore tends to be less frequently positive and more frequently intense. Interpersonal difficulties would appear to be more acute for them. The relationship tends to be intense but often involves conflicts, and the tensions involved are uncertain, poorly controlled, and out of keeping with the environment. Among the prepared women, on the other hand, we find a kind of 'normalization' of the relationship. If preparation improves the adjustment of the woman to the staff, it is by stemming the manifestations of tensions and conflicts and creating a kind of fixed and well-maintained distance. It must, however, be noted that the relationship is not thereby rendered overwhelmingly positive, since the frequency of ambivalent relationships remains the same, and is as high as that of positive relationships; and, when the relationship is positive, it tends to be not particularly intense.

These results raise the question of what in fact constitutes a 'good relationship'. In the previous chapter, it was emphasized that assessment is relative to a definite frame of reference with its own standards. Thus, within the frame of reference of the PPM, a good relationship is no doubt this relationship at an appropriate distance, which tends to appear among prepared women. But it is clear that a good relationship might be defined differently in a different frame of reference. In particular, more direct consideration might be taken of its transference significance, or of its value as a maturing experience and so on. But the use of such a frame of reference would have been justified only if a clinical approach at a deeper level had been adopted.

Let us now consider how relations with staff are associated with the other confinement variables. In order to calculate the relevant correlations, it was necessary to combine quality and intensity into a single dimension, since neither could be treated separately for the purpose of statistical analysis, the interpretation of each depending upon the other. The nine categories were reduced to a four-point relationship scale, in such a way as to be as far as possible in line with clinical impressions:

Category 1: good relationship – positive relationship of strong or average intensity;

Category 2: average relationship – positive but weak relationship, or ambivalent relationship of weak or average intensity;

Category 3: poor relationship – strong ambivalent relationship;

Category 4: very poor relationship – negative relationship, regardless of intensity.

Table 10 gives the correlations between this global score of relationship to staff and the confinement scores. It shows that the quality of the relationship is significantly related to the success of the confinement. The correlation for prepared women is 0·45, and, in this group,

TABLE 10   CORRELATIONS BETWEEN RELATIONS WITH
STAFF AND CONFINEMENT SCORES

		1 *Dila-* *tation*	*Stages* *2* *Trans-* *ition*	*3* *Expul-* *sion*	*4* *Issue*	*Stages combined* *1 + 2*	*3 + 4*	*Total*
Pain	PPM	+·27	+·23	+·21	+·18	+·29	+·28	+·31
	U	(+·48)	(+·45)	(+·51)	(+·49)	(+·50)	(+·58)	(+·69)
Behaviour	PPM	+·34	+·41	+·47	+·33	+·41	+·43	+·50
	U	(+·60)	(+·53)	(+·55)	(+·62)	(+·60)	(+·65)	(+·73)
Total	PPM	+·32	+·41	+·43	+·26	+·39	+·37	+·45
	U	(+·63)	(+·56)	(+·59)	(+·61)	(+·64)	(+·51)	(+·80)

the correlation with behavioural control (0·50) is greater than that with pain (0·31). Among unprepared women, the correlation between relations with staff and success of confinement is 0·80, and, in this group, the correlations with behavioural control and with pain are roughly the same (0·73 with behavioural control and 0·69 with pain).

Before an overall interpretation of the results concerning relationship with staff can be arrived at, several findings must be considered.

In the first place, good relationships with staff are found more frequently among prepared women than among unprepared women. Several factors seem to be involved here. The prepared women are, to some extent, pre-adjusted to the obstetrical staff; they are therefore in a better position to feel confidence in the staff and to establish good mutual relations. Again, women who have chosen preparation are, in general, women who are better adjusted socially, as will be shown in the next chapter. Factors connected with the selection and composition of the two groups are therefore added to those deriving directly from preparation. These differences between the groups in respect of their interpersonal adjustment, which can be traced right through the lives of the members and particularly during pregnancy, naturally tend to find expression during confinement itself. Moreover, the obstetrical staff themselves no doubt tend to establish different relationships with the women, according to whether or not they have been prepared. When women prepared by the PPM are involved, the interpersonal field is better defined, and, as it were, 'normalized' by the implicit adoption of criteria common to both midwives and parturients, and so the probability of harmonious interaction is increased. When unprepared women are involved, the relationship is much more strongly saturated with transference and counter-transference factors that appear spontaneously during the meeting. The attitude of midwives towards unprepared women varies quite a lot: sometimes it is rather hostile; sometimes, on the other hand, it is especially favourable and gratifying when the woman behaves well in spite of not being prepared. Clearly, our statistical approach is not capable of unravelling all these interrelated factors.

In the second place, a good relationship with the staff is closely connected with the general success of the confinement, and here, of course, we have a case of mutual causality. A good relationship no doubt favours a good confinement, but, conversely, a good relationship can also be more easily established the more smoothly the

129

confinement proceeds. It does appear, however, in a clinical assessment of childbirth, that a good relationship is more frequently cause than effect. The notion can, in any case, be retained as a hypothesis.

A third point is that the association between relations with staff and the overall success of the confinement is closer for unprepared women than for prepared women. We previously saw that relations with the staff were more 'significant' for unprepared women than for prepared women; that is, they expressed more directly the transference conflicts associated with deep-lying anxieties. It would therefore appear that relations with staff are more closely associated with the success of the confinement when they are more significant, or more specifically determined by the whole personality of the woman. This is no doubt why we find that the relationship with the staff, among unprepared women, is closely associated not only with behavioural adjustment but also with pain, that is, it operates at the level of the most deep-lying anxiety; whereas, among prepared women, this association is more superficial and concerns mainly behavioural control.

It cannot, therefore, be too strongly emphasized that the relationship with the staff is an individual psychological variable which is of particular importance in childbirth. It undoubtedly represents one of the main variables to be taken into account in defining a 'good confinement' in terms which go beyond the simple quantitative assessment of behavioural control and analgesia.

RELATION TO THE BABY

The relation to the baby was assessed with respect to quality and intensity in the same way as were relations with the staff. In this case, the intention was to evaluate the reaction of the mother to the first contact with her baby. The procedure was meant to be more intuitive than descriptive here. It was hoped, in particular, to isolate the quality of affect expressed in spontaneous verbalization or, in the absence of any verbalization, by gestures, signs, and other expressions.

As far as the comparison of prepared and unprepared women is concerned, *Table 11* shows somewhat different results with respect to the quality and intensity of the relation to the baby from those reported for relations with the staff. In this case, the prepared women show a clear preponderance of positive relationships (56 per cent).

TABLE 11   DISTRIBUTION OF PREPARED AND UNPREPARED
WOMEN WITH RESPECT TO INTENSITY AND QUALITY OF
RELATION TO BABY

Quality		Strong	Intensity Average	Weak	Total
		%	%	%	%
Positive	PPM	27	25	4	56
	U	(0)	(12)	(4)	(16)
Ambivalent	PPM	11	9	14	34
	U	(23)	(15)	(27)	(65)
Negative	PPM	2	6	2	10
	U	(4)	(7·5)	(7·5)	(19)
Total	PPM	40	40	20	
	U	(27)	(34·5)	(38·5)	

For the unprepared women, on the other hand, positive relationships are relatively rare and it is ambivalent relationships that predominate, even more clearly here than in the case of relations with the staff, which also showed a relative predominance of ambivalent relationships. The difference between the two groups is thus more marked for relationship to the baby than for relationship with the staff.

Here again, it may be wondered how far this difference is due to the effects of preparation and how far to personality factors which vary between the groups, and one can but note the interaction between these different kinds of factors.

The correlations between relation to the child and confinement scores are given in *Table 12*. On the whole, they are lower than those involving relations with the staff. One point in particular stands out

131

TABLE 12   CORRELATIONS BETWEEN RELATION TO BABY
AND CONFINEMENT SCORES

| | | | *Stages* | | | *Stages combined* | | |
		1	*2*	*3*	*4*	*1 + 2*	*3 + 4*	*Total*
Pain	PPM	+·17	+·21	+·23	+·22	+·22	+·18	+·27
	U	(+·16)	(+·27)	(+·02)	(−·14)	(+·25)	(−·08)	(+·10)
Behaviour	PPM	+·21	+·20	+·41	+·33	+·23	+·39	+·32
	U	(+·25)	(+·50)	(+·47)	(+·37)	(+·40)	(+·46)	(+·51)
Total	PPM	+·21	+·23	+·34	+·31	+·24	+·35	+·35
	U	(+·25)	(+·44)	(+·35)	(+·09)	(+·39)	(+·33)	(+·38)

in *Table 12*: whereas, among the prepared women, the correlations
with pain and with behavioural control are about the same, among
the unprepared women, the correlation with behavioural control is
quite clear (0·51), while that with pain is negligible (0·10).

This last finding did not appear with regard to relations with the
staff. Relations with the staff were closely associated with both pain
and behaviour among the unprepared women, whereas the relation to
the baby appears to be particularly associated with behavioural
control.

Furthermore, although there is an appreciable correlation between
relations with the staff and relationship to the baby, this is not nearly as
large as might have been expected (0·39 among prepared women, 0·33
among unprepared women). It follows that certain determinants or
aspects of confinement may be more specifically associated with
relations with the staff and others with the relation to the baby.

It may be of interest to try to reinterpret these results in such a way
as to integrate both relations with the staff and relation to the baby.
The patterns that emerge are clearly different, and even contrasted,
according to whether prepared or unprepared women are
concerned.

132

Among unprepared women, relations with the staff are closely associated with both pain and behavioural control; on the other hand, relation to the baby is associated only with behavioural control. It may be that a very positive maternal attitude is a factor in behavioural adjustment during confinement, which enables the anxieties specific to childbirth to be masked or even overcome by a kind of current adjustment, while these anxieties nevertheless find expression at a deeper level in the form of pain. For anxiety to be genuinely overcome at all levels, the personality of the woman must be such as will enable her to establish positive relationships with the staff. Only when this is so will she be able to achieve a measure of analgesia.

Among women prepared by the PPM, behavioural control is associated, though less markedly, with both relations with the staff and relation to the baby. These correlations indicate that these women show a kind of neutralized and normalized behaviour, which includes among its norms certain 'ideal types' of relations with the staff and relation to the baby. The relations themselves are thus actually improved, but lose something of their personal significance as criteria of a good confinement.

It must be added that the relation to the baby, to which special importance has been attached in our research hypotheses, has in fact been assessed only in a relatively superficial manner. The assessment was based upon the first reactions of the woman during the moments immediately following the birth. This moment in time may well be of less critical significance than we have been inclined to believe, and it may be possible to assess the real quality of the relation to the baby only by continuing observation during the hours and days following the birth. The limited nature of our assessment therefore enjoins caution in generalizing the results obtained on this question.

EFFECTS OF PPM TECHNIQUES

The effects of the PPM have been frequently referred to in the foregoing analyses of results. It has, however, been emphasized repeatedly that the observed differences between the prepared and the unprepared women could not all be attributed to preparation itself. Indeed, as will appear in the succeeding chapters, the two groups of women differ considerably in various aspects of their past history and in various personality characteristics, which are themselves partly

133

responsible for the acceptance or rejection of preparation. Accordingly, it may be of greater value to try to assess the differential effects of preparation within the prepared group itself.

An assessment of the use of PPM techniques during confinement, which was intended to be as objective and exact as possible, was included in the design of our research. The techniques involved are of three kinds:

(a) The breathing technique consists in the adoption of certain breathing rhythms at different stages during labour: full, deep breathing to accompany the slow rhythm of the first uterine contractions; rapid, superficial breathing to match the faster rhythm of the uterine contractions at the end of labour; panting during the transition phase; and, finally, holding of the breath followed by expiration to facilitate bearing down.

(b) The relaxation technique consists in an attempt to achieve neuromuscular relaxation both during dilatation and during birth.

(c) The technique of bearing down is intended to secure effective and rapid expulsive efforts and to facilitate the maximum degree of participation in the birth.

The aim of our assessment was to quantify two dimensions: the extent to which the techniques were employed, on the one hand, and their efficacy, on the other. The ratings for the employment of the techniques were made in terms of the usual standards, according to the criteria explained to the women when they were learning the techniques. A well-executed breathing movement was scored 1; if it was performed in a very unskilled and inappropriate way it was scored 3; and if it fell between these two extremes it was scored 2. The effectiveness of the techniques was assessed in a different way. The main basis for the assessment was the woman's immediate opinion as to the help that she thought any of the techniques had provided during labour, and her own view of their analgesic effects. Her account during the post-confinement interview was also taken into consideration.

The correlations presented in *Table 13* and discussed below were calculated from a composite score, combining the scores for employment and for effectiveness of the techniques, but giving more weight to employment as being the more objective assessment.

It will be seen, from *Table 13,* that the correlations between the global confinement scores and the technique scores are quite high (0·63, 0·60, and 0·69); in other words, the more adequately the

TABLE 13   CORRELATIONS BETWEEN USE OF PPM TECHNIQUES (BREATHING, RELAXATION, BEARING DOWN) AND CONFINEMENT SCORES

		Stages 1	2	3	4	Stages combined 1 + 2	3 + 4	Total
	a	+·58	+·48	+·31	+·14	+·59	+·16	+·54
Pain	b	+·47	+·36	+·30	+·25	+·47	+·24	+·50
	c	+·02	+·15	+·30	+·45	+·09	+·39	+·27
	a	+·63	+·58	+·46	+·24	+·66	+·37	+·56
Behaviour	b	+·53	+·51	+·46	+·33	+·56	+·42	+·52
	c	+·17	+·17	+·53	+·51	+·19	+·56	+·41
	a	+·57	+·60	+·47	+·19	+·69	+·35	+·63
Total	b	+·54	+·52	+·47	+·33	+·57	+·43	+·60
	c	+·09	+·21	+·47	+·44	+·16	+·50	+·69

a = breathing; b = relaxation; c = bearing down

techniques are applied, the more successful will be the confinement, and vice versa. This is scarcely surprising, and only confirms the positive role of good preparation for a successful confinement, which a considerable number of studies have already demonstrated.

A study of the correlations between the different techniques and the different stages of the confinement shows some interesting features. Breathing has more effect during the dilatation-transition stage than during expulsion-issue, and the same is true for relaxation, although less clearly so. Bearing down is significantly correlated with confinement only during expulsion-issue, since it is only then that it is involved. We might, indeed, have expected this correlation to be higher, the technique of bearing down being functionally integrated into the process of labour itself; but it should be stressed that the technique of bearing down is very difficult to assess and, accordingly, too much significance should not be attached to this result.

With regard to their effects on behaviour and pain, respectively, it is clear that the techniques – whether of breathing or of relaxation – during the first main stage affect behaviour and pain equally; during the second main stage, however, they exert a more marked effect on behaviour than on pain.

Correlations between the techniques themselves were also calculated. A positive correlation of 0·63 was found between breathing and relaxation, but no significant correlation emerged between either of these two techniques and bearing down.

It also seemed interesting to see how far the use of the techniques was related to initial motivation for accepting preparation. An estimate of motivation, both deep-lying and superficial, as expressed by the woman with regard to the PPM, was therefore sought in the case-histories. Three degrees of motivation were distinguished, according to whether the views expressed appeared to be valid and genuinely held (1), or ambivalent (2), or simply superficial rationalizations of a choice in which there was little involvement (3). It may be that there are women in the third of these groups who choose preparation without any genuine motivation, and who in effect deny themselves the right to believe in the possibility of obstetrical analgesia.

Our results indicate that too much significance should not be attached to the initial motivation of the women for accepting the PPM. *Table 14* shows that such correlation as exists between motivation and the quality of the confinement is not very high, and involves behaviour rather than pain. The motivated women are conscientious

TABLE 14 CORRELATIONS BETWEEN MOTIVA-
TION FOR PPM AND CONFINEMENT SCORES

| | *Stages* | | |
	1 + 2	*3 + 4*	*Total*
Pain	+·18	+·25	+·22
Behaviour	+·31	+·26	+·33
Total	+·28	+·23	+·31

during their period of instruction, and show themselves to be apt pupils; they tend to show behaviour that is well adjusted to the situation about which they have been instructed, and hence tend to show positive results in terms of behaviour without this necessarily being accompanied by any real analgesia.

There is a relationship between motivation to accept preparation and the use of the techniques during confinement, but this is lower than might have been expected (about 0·35). It must therefore be concluded that the effective application of the method learned depends on a considerable number of factors which modify the effect of the initial motivation.

In the standard theory of the PPM, activity is a notion closely connected with the actual practice of the techniques learned. It therefore seemed of interest to see whether our results revealed any correlations between the activity score and the technique scores. The correlations were in fact 0·27 with breathing, 0·32 with relaxation, and 0·46 with bearing down. Bearing down is therefore the technique which is most closely associated with activity. A significant correlation between activity and bearing down might certainly have been anticipated; but a sizable correlation might also have been expected between activity and breathing. The results here obtained are without any doubt explicable in terms of the particular definition of activity adopted in the present research, which differs appreciably from its usual definition in works on the PPM; and no doubt it is at the moment of the birth itself that the technique learned calls for the greatest degree of direct deep 'involvement' in the course of the confinement.

Finally, *Table 15* shows that there is also a correlation between the use of the techniques and both relations with the staff and relation to the baby. These correlations are relatively small. It does seem, nevertheless, that the use of the techniques must continually interact with the relations that develop in the labour ward between the parturient woman and the hospital staff. The woman is naturally sustained in her use of the techniques by the instructions and encouragement provided by the staff, and, reciprocally, good use of the techniques is bound to encourage cooperation and the establishment of positive relationships. It is, accordingly, the smallness of the observed correlation that appears surprising. This should serve to emphasize yet further the complex nature of the interpersonal processes involved in confinement, processes in which both immediate and situational factors on

TABLE 15 CORRELATIONS BETWEEN USE OF
PPM TECHNIQUES AND RELATIONS WITH
STAFF AND TO BABY

Use of techniques	*Relations with staff*	*Relation to baby*
Breathing	+·29	+·22
Relaxation	+·36	+·31
Bearing down	+·34	+·23

the one hand, and factors concerned with personal history and transference on the other, are constantly interacting.

SUMMARY

An examination of the distribution of the global confinement scores shows that these discriminate effectively between the women, and that a genuine 'psychometric variable' is involved. The separate scores for pain and behavioural control appear to be comparable in size and to contribute about equally to the total score. Similarly, the two main stages into which the confinements were divided for the purpose of recording observations (dilatation-transition and expulsion-issue) contribute approximately equally to the total. The importance of pain, however, seems to decrease from the first stage to the second.

Women prepared by the PPM have better confinements. In particular, their behavioural control is better than that of unprepared women. If the difference between behavioural control score and pain score (for each case) is taken as an index of 'level of control', it appears that this index is significantly more positive among prepared women. It also appears that improvement due to preparation is more marked during the dilatation-transition stage than during the expulsion-issue stage.

True obstetrical factors appear to be of relatively little importance. It must, however, be emphasized that, in the sample population, only

138

minor incidents were involved (use of drugs, prolonged labour, etc.), all cases involving more serious incidents (e.g. forceps delivery) having been eliminated. Even so, it was found that an abnormally long labour raised the pain score and increased the probability of disorganization of behaviour during the dilatation-transition stage.

More important appear to be the 'qualitative' aspects of confinement which were separately recorded and scored. Activity, defined as a kind of 'global level of involvement in the situation', on average was as high among unprepared as among prepared women. On the other hand, relations with the staff of the labour ward and the first relation to the baby were significantly better in prepared women. For both prepared and unprepared women, these two factors are significantly related to the success of the confinement. Good relations with the staff, however, are most clearly associated with a good confinement in the case of unprepared women. Thus, although preparation improves this relationship as a whole, a good 'spontaneous' relationship is still, for unprepared women, a quite significant indicator of those aspects of personality and those attitudes that are conducive to a good confinement.

Beyond the purely statistical analysis, consideration of these qualitative aspects of confinement appears fundamental for understanding the individual dynamics which, in each case, underlie the woman's personal reaction to her confinement, its more or less favourable development, and the success or failure of the psychological analgesia associated with the PPM.

In themselves, the various ways we have put forward for assessing confinements constitute a systematic method for the collection, classification, and evaluation of data – a rich method, and one that is effective in revealing the individual structures that underlie these dynamics.

Finally, it should be noted that, when the various correlations are examined in detail, the observed relationships are rather different among prepared and unprepared women, for reasons which are often difficult to analyse, and which consequently suggest the need for more detailed research in this field.

G. GAYLE STEPHENS, M.D.
3232 East Pine
Wichita, Kansas   67208

CHAPTER 7

Negativity

Negative Factors in the Woman's Physical and Psychological History

---

Having examined the confinement scores, we now turn to consider the negativity scores for our experimental groups.

The negativity scores, which will be correlated with the confinement scores, vary from one woman to another according to a number of factors which have to be controlled before the obtained correlations can be correctly interpreted. Moreover, it is possible that the two groups, prepared and unprepared, differ significantly in negativity, and any such differences must be known if the combined effects of negativity and preparation upon confinement are to be explained. Finally, the internal structure of the measuring instrument must itself be demonstrated by the obtained results if the significance of the measures it provides is to be properly understood.

GLOBAL INDICES OF NEGATIVITY

If we examine the distribution of global negativity scores for the whole experimental population, including both prepared and unprepared women, we find that it approximates a normal distribution (*Figure 3*). This tends to show that the negativity grid discriminates satisfactorily between subjects. It also contributes towards the validation of the operational concept of negativity as defined in the present study by showing that such a concept does provide the basis of a significant individual variable in terms of which subjects are normally distributed. If, however, we examine the prepared women and the unprepared women separately, we find that the distributions of global negativity scores are appreciably different for the two groups (*Figure 4*). The distribution of scores for the prepared women is very similar to that for the total sample, being only slightly skewed towards the low

140

Figure 3   Distribution of global negativity scores for 116 women (90 prepared, 26 unprepared)

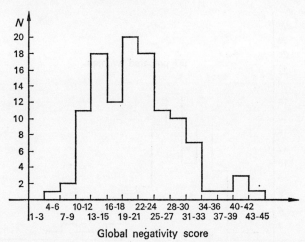

Global negativity score

negativity end. The distribution for the unprepared women, on the other hand, does not approximate the normal curve but more closely resembles a bimodal distribution, with the main peak towards the high negativity end and a smaller peak towards the low negativity end.

This observation is reflected in a comparison of the mean scores of the two groups, which are 20·44 for the prepared women and 23·54 for the unprepared women. This difference is significant at about the 0·05 level.

A first examination of the global negativity scores thus indicates a difference between the prepared and the unprepared women, and this difference will have to be taken into consideration when the relations between negativity and confinement in the two groups are investigated. Independently of the effects of preparation, which differentiate the two groups with respect to quality of confinement, we cannot ignore the fact that there is an initial difference between the two groups.

This difference may not be unconnected with choice or refusal of preparation. The women who choose to be prepared by the PPM tend on average to be well-adjusted women with fewer personal difficulties. The most plausible hypothesis is that their confinement is likely to be better both because of their better initial adjustment and because of

141

Figure 4   Distribution of global negativity scores for 90 prepared women
and for 26 unprepared women

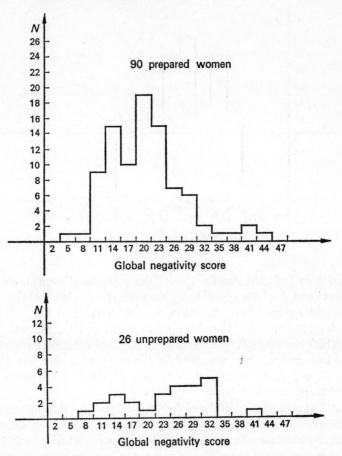

the benefits of preparation; but, to establish this hypothesis, we need
to know with respect to which aspects of negativity the two groups are
most clearly distinguished. The rest of this chapter will be devoted to a
study of the results obtained when the various aspects of negativity
are taken separately, according to stages and areas. This analysis is
essential if we are to understand the meaning of the global index
itself, and will also enable us to specify in detail the aspects in which the
two groups differ.

142

ANALYSIS OF NEGATIVITY BY PERIODS

NEGATIVITY I (IN PERSONAL HISTORY) AND NEGATIVITY II
(DURING PREGNANCY)

Table 16 shows that the number of negative factors recorded is
different in the two main parts of the grid. It is, on average, significantly higher for the first part than for the second part. This is obviously

TABLE 16   MEANS AND STANDARD DEVIATIONS OF NEGATIVITY
SCORES

		Prepared group	Unprepared group	t
Negativity I	m	12·93	14·15	0·90 n.s.
	σ	6·05	6·30	
Negativity II	m	7·59	9·38	2·19 ·02 < p < ·05
	σ	3·53	4·12	
Total negativity	m	20·44	23·54	1·83 ·05 < p < ·10
	σ	7·44	8·10	

connected with the way in which the grid is constructed: one is clearly
more likely to obtain a large number of negativity entries when the
constituent elements on which the entries are based are more numerous
or more detailed. This does not entitle us to draw any conclusions
about the relative importance of the negative factors in the two main
periods. But the weight given to the first period relative to the second
in the actual structure of the grid plainly reflects the significance that
we wished to attach to the influence of factors in the past histories of
the parturient women. Negativity in the personal history was emphasized for several reasons. First, in view of our theoretical outlook, we
tended to attach a high degree of influence to past experience and to

look for the origins of current problems or conflicts in the whole life-history of the woman. Second, the prominence of the first part of the grid was a consequence of the relatively long period of time which it covered compared with the short duration of pregnancy.

The comparison of prepared and unprepared women in the two parts of the grid confirms that unprepared women tend to show more negativity, both in their personal histories and during pregnancy. The difference between the groups is, however, more significant for negativity during pregnancy. This suggests, on the one hand, that negative factors in the woman's past history may contribute to the refusal of preparation by the PPM, but, on the other hand, that the absence of preparation tends to reinforce the effects of this pre-existing negativity on negativity during pregnancy itself. In other words, it would seem that preparation is of definite help during pregnancy, tending to reduce the incidence of anxiety and conflict. This finding, which has very important practical implications, needs to be confirmed by a more detailed analysis of the factors of negativity which appear in the two groups of prepared and unprepared women during pregnancy.

The significance of the total negativity score is elucidated by an examination of the correlations between the partial totals for the two main periods and the overall total. These correlations indicate the weight of the two main periods in the total. *Table 17* shows that the first part of the negativity grid contributes more to this total. The

TABLE 17 CORRELATIONS BETWEEN NEGATIVITY I (IN PERSONAL HISTORY), NEGATIVITY II (DURING PREGNANCY), AND TOTAL NEGATIVITY

		Negativity II	*Total negativity*
Negativity I	PPM	+·28	+·90
	U	(+·17)	(+·86)
Negativity II	PPM		+·65
	U		(+·64)

correlations of the first part with the total (0·90 and 0·86) actually suggest that a sufficiently accurate estimate of total negativity could be obtained from the first part only. It is, however, an advantage to retain the information provided by the second part of the grid. This introduces an additional factor differentiating between the women. The correlations between the two parts of the grid are, in fact, remarkably low (0·28 for prepared women and 0·17 for unprepared women). The inclusion of factors connected with negativity during pregnancy in the total thus contributes new material of a very different kind from that contributed by negativity in the personal history. The addition of these two should therefore give a more comprehensive idea of the actual disadvantages under which each woman is suffering. It should also be observed that the correlations to which we have just referred are of comparable size in both groups of women. This suggests that the negativity grid is a reliable instrument, measuring on the whole the same kinds of facts, whatever the particular characteristics of the groups involved.

ANALYSIS OF NEGATIVITY BY MORE FINELY DELIMITED
PERIODS

The chronological breakdown of the factors of negativity included in the grid enables us to analyse in greater detail the relative importance of the data collected for the different periods and the respective contribution made by each period to the total negativity score. If we examine the three periods making up the first part of the grid (negativity in the personal history: childhood, adolescence, and adulthood), we find, as *Table 18* shows, that the amount of information collected increases from childhood to adolescence and from adolescence to adulthood. This is so for both prepared and unprepared women. Here again, it is difficult to distinguish what is due to the structure of the grid from what is due to the nature of the facts themselves. One point, however, suggests that the structure of the grid cannot be the only factor. The way the questions were defined tended to involve a lot of itemization of material for the childhood period. In particular, anything concerned with family life during childhood and with interpersonal relations within the family is likely to be noted in great detail. It is perhaps surprising, therefore, that this period supplies so few entries, especially when a whole section of the first interview was

145

TABLE 18 MEANS AND STANDARD DEVIATIONS OF
NEGATIVITY SCORES BY PERIODS

Period		Prepared group	Unprepared group	t
Ia	m	3·16	3·12	n.s.
Childhood	σ	2·62	2·85	
Ib	m	4·17	4·54	n.s.
Adolescence	σ	2·59	2·91	
Ic	m	5·59	6·50	1·12
Adulthood	σ	3·61	3·87	n.s.
IIa	m	3·70	4·85	2·30
First stage of				$·02 < p < ·05$
pregnancy	σ	2·13	2·60	
IIb	m	3·96	4·54	1·09
Second stage of				n.s.
pregnancy	σ	2·42	2·26	

devoted to surveying childhood and listing factors concerning family
background; the women were thus specifically invited to recall events,
conflicts, and traumatic incidents relating to this period. It would in
fact appear that a very important proximity factor is involved here: the
women tend particularly to quote current or very recent events rather
than those that took place a long time ago. It is therefore to adulthood that the women refer most frequently when discussing their
problems or their conflicts. To this pure and simple effect of proximity,
which naturally tends to favour reference to recent events, are no doubt
added effects specifically related to the dynamics of past experience –
amnesia concerning childhood, and a tendency to rationalization in
the present. It should also be noted that the period of adolescence

evokes a greater number of important events than does the rest of childhood, although chronologically it is relatively short. Here again, no doubt the proximity factor is involved; but we must also remember that adolescence is a particularly critical period, and therefore essentially productive of conflict. The new crisis represented by pregnancy may in fact tend to revive the conflicts experienced during adolescence. In this case, there would be a kind of meaningful continuity between adolescence and pregnancy. This, which appears clearly to be the case for unconscious processes, would also be true for spontaneous reference to events and current rationalizations, and would thus be reflected in our system of scoring.

Finally, if we examine negativity during pregnancy as a whole, little difference is to be found between the two stages of pregnancy in respect of the number of negative items. The difference between the two groups of prepared and unprepared women, which, for the whole period of pregnancy, indicated that the unprepared women showed significantly greater negativity, remains constant throughout pregnancy and is no more related to one period than to the other.

CORRELATIONS BETWEEN DIFFERENT PERIODS OF NEGATIVITY

In this analysis of negativity by periods, there remains to be considered the relative weight of the five periods distinguished in the global index of negativity. *Table 19* gives the correlations of each of the partial scores for these periods with the total negativity score, for prepared and unprepared women respectively. For both groups of women, the largest contribution to the total negativity score is made by the negative elements in the period of adulthood preceding pregnancy (0·73 and 0·72 respectively). Among prepared women, this is followed, in order of importance, by later pregnancy and adolescence, with childhood and early pregnancy coming last. Among unprepared women, the order of importance is different: apart from the predominating influence of adulthood, all the other periods seem to have roughly equal weight in the total negativity score.

The most marked difference between the groups concerns the respective contributions of the two stages of pregnancy. As we have seen, among prepared women, the same *number* of negative items was found in both stages of pregnancy, and this was also the

TABLE 19 INTERCORRELATIONS BETWEEN NEGATIVITY
SCORES (BY PERIODS, PARTIAL TOTALS, GRAND TOTAL)

		Ia	Ib	Ic	N I	IIa	IIb	N II
Ib	PPM	+·18						
	U	(+·27)						
Ic	PPM	+·08	+·32					
	U	(+·08)	(+·09)					
N I	PPM	+·56	+·70	+·77				
	U	(+·62)	(+·64)	(+·68)				
IIa	PPM	−·07	−·02	+·24	+·10			
	U	(+·01)	(−·19)	(+·41)	(+·37)			
IIb	PPM	+·13	+·19	+·36	+·36	+·17		
	U	(+·01)	(−·01)	(+·20)	(+·12)	(+·44)		
N II	PPM	·00	+·10	+·39	+·28	+·71	+·79	
	U	(·00)	(−·13)	(+·37)	(+·17)	(+·87)	(+·82)	
T N	PPM	+·47	+·61	+·73	+·90	+·38	+·63	+·65
	U	(+·48)	(+·43)	(+·72)	(+·86)	(+·57)	(+·51)	(+·64)

Ia = childhood
Ib = adolescence
Ic = adulthood
N I = total negativity in personal
       history

IIa = first stage of pregnancy
IIb = second stage of pregnancy
N II = total negativity during preg-
        nancy
T N = total negativity (I + II)

case for unprepared women. But among the prepared women the
negative items in the second stage, although not more numerous,
contribute significantly more to the total than do the items in the first
stage (correlations of 0·63 and 0·38 respectively). For the unprepared

women, on the other hand, the contributions of the two stages of pregnancy to the total negativity score are approximately equal (correlations of 0·51 and 0·57 respectively).

To throw light on the somewhat complex significance of these findings, let us consider the intercorrelations between the stages themselves. *Table 19* also gives these figures. On the whole, the childhood period has the lowest correlations with the other periods, for both prepared and unprepared women. There is an appreciable correlation (0·32) between adolescence and adulthood, but only for prepared women. Further, for prepared women, adulthood is also correlated with the two stages of pregnancy, the correlation with the second stage being higher than that with the first stage. This is reversed in the case of unprepared women, for whom the only period showing an appreciable correlation with adult negativity is the first stage of pregnancy (0·41). The correlation between the two stages of pregnancy themselves is significantly higher for unprepared women than for prepared women. It is not easy to bring these various findings into a coherent and meaningful pattern. The most striking thing is that the intercorrelations are so different for prepared and unprepared women. Childhood negativity alone is relatively unconnected with negativity in the other periods in both groups of women; but, for all the other periods, the relationships frequently tend to be somewhat contradictory in the two groups.

The only relatively consistent finding is that negativity in previous adult life and negativity during pregnancy are related. As far as the prepared women are concerned, it is not difficult to understand how the effects of adult negativity tend to be greater during the second stage of pregnancy than during the first stage. The acceptance of preparation may itself provide, at the beginning of pregnancy, a form of reassurance against anxiety which tends to mask the effects of the earlier negativity. But as the confinement comes near, this reassurance becomes progressively less effective, paradoxically just when preparation is becoming effective. As far as the unprepared women are concerned, on the other hand, it is at the beginning of pregnancy that anxiety is most closely related to pre-existing disabilities and, in particular, to any disturbing experience in the adult period immediately preceding pregnancy. But it is difficult to explain why this relationship should become weaker in the second stage of pregnancy, especially in view of the fact that, among unprepared women, there is an appreciable

correlation between the two stages of pregnancy in respect of negativity (0·44), while this correlation is much lower among prepared
women (0·17). In the present state of our knowledge, a satisfactory
answer to this problem, which would resolve this apparent contradiction, seems impossible. This somewhat paradoxical finding would
have to be integrated with the other finding, referred to above, that the
difference between prepared and unprepared women with respect to
anxiety directly concerned with pregnancy and confinement is more
marked in the first stage of pregnancy than in the second stage. On the
whole, the results seem to suggest that negativity during the second
stage of pregnancy is relatively unpredictable in unprepared women,
since it is not clearly related to negativity in any of the other periods.

To summarize, the study of negativity by periods yields results
which are difficult to interpret as a whole and in which the effects of
preparation are not clearly apparent.

ANALYSIS OF NEGATIVITY BY AREAS

NEGATIVITY IN TWELVE AREAS

We shall first of all examine, as in the case of our analysis by periods,
the number of negativity entries in the different areas represented in
the grid.

Table 20 gives the means and standard deviations of the partial
negativity scores according to area, for negativity in the personal
history and for negativity during pregnancy respectively. As far as
negativity in the personal history is concerned, the areas of womanhood (B) and interpersonal disturbances (C) contain the largest
number of negative items. For negativity during pregnancy, the
negative items are more evenly distributed over the different areas.
Here, the only area in which there is an especially large number of
negative items is the area of psychopathological symptoms relating to
pregnancy (E), in which are included all the anxieties and fears
directly connected with pregnancy and childbirth.

The comparison of prepared and unprepared women in the different
areas of negativity yields particularly interesting results. The difference
found between the global negativity scores of the two groups is not
reflected equally in each area, but is derived particularly from certain
areas.

150

TABLE 20 MEANS AND STANDARD DEVIATIONS BY
AREAS OF NEGATIVITY

Area		Prepared group	Unprepared group	t
NEGATIVITY I				
A Individual pathology	m	2·22	1·62	1·49
	σ	1·87	1·55	n.s.
B Womanhood	m	4·18	3·96	0·04
	σ	2·43	2·53	n.s.
C Family background	m	5·69	7·58	2·12
	σ	3·78	4·67	·02 < p < ·05
D Social life	m	0·81	1·00	n.s.
	σ	0·96	1·21	
NEGATIVITY II				
A General pathology	m	0·44	0·65	1·44
	σ	0·67	0·62	n.s.
B Gynaeco-obstetrical	m	0·37	0·23	n.s.
pathology	σ	0·82	0·50	
C Psychosomatic symptoms	m	1·10	1·23	n.s.
specific to pregnancy	σ	1·02	0·89	
D Abnormalities in	m	0·83	0·69	n.s.
maternal attitude	σ	1·10	0·95	
E Psychopathological	m	2·83	3·15	n.s.
symptoms (anxieties)	σ	1·76	1·70	
F Personality and	m	0·48	0·46	n.s.
behaviour disorders	σ	0·73	0·80	
G Family problems	m	0·81	1·92	3·36
	σ	1·13	2·40	p = ·001
H Social difficulties	m	0·77	1·03	1·30
	σ	0·93	0·81	n.s.

In the first part of the grid, it is essentially in area C, interpersonal disturbances, that the unprepared women show, on average, a higher level of negativity than do prepared women. In area B, womanhood, there is no appreciable difference between the groups. In area D, social difficulties, the difference is also very small, although it suggests

151

that such difficulties may perhaps be a little less frequent for the prepared women. On the other hand, in area A, which includes all pathological indications existing before pregnancy, the mean negativity score is higher for the prepared than for the unprepared women.

For the first part of the grid, representing negativity in the personal history prior to pregnancy, the differences in disabilities between the two groups probably reflect the factors that influence acceptance or refusal of preparation. Thus, women who refuse preparation are characterized particularly by a greater frequency of conflicts in relation to their families. In this group of women, we find, on the one hand, a greater frequency of negative family incidents in their past experience and, on the other, a general tendency to develop conflict-laden relationships in the immediate environment, although these relationships are not directed exclusively towards a particular person in this environment. There would appear to be little doubt that the existence of these family problems tends to constitute an obstacle to choosing to be prepared by the PPM. In contrast, motives for refusing preparation seem to bear no relation to the problems of womanhood, as might have been expected. Finally, the existence of major pathological factors in earlier life would tend rather to increase the likelihood of accepting preparation. This finding can be interpreted in different ways: on the one hand, a kind of sensitization to illness might induce the women, at the beginning of their pregnancy, to be more afraid of possible complications and to seek protection by joining a group offering security; on the other hand, a greater familiarity with hospital or medical circles might make them more ready to apply to them for help.

A characteristic picture thus emerges of certain women who refuse preparation: women who, after a rather disturbed family life, find it difficult to establish new relationships or who establish, in the manner of a transference, disturbed relationships with those with whom they are currently in contact, and are consequently hostile to any involvement in a new interpersonal context; women particularly inclined to develop defensive attitudes, who tend to deny the anxieties evoked by pregnancy and try to regard it as a very ordinary event, especially if they themselves are in good health.

The differences between the two groups of women in respect of negativity during pregnancy are slight. The only marked differences

152

are in areas G and H, which cover respectively interpersonal disturbances in the family situation and difficulties in social adjustment.
Unprepared women score higher in both of these, which is in line with
the greater frequency of family problems in their past life, already
referred to.

It is rather surprising to find that preparation itself does not seem
to have much effect upon the experience of pregnancy. We previously
noted that prepared and unprepared women differed little with respect
to past development of womanhood, and we now find that their
attitudes to womanhood and motherhood differ little during pregnancy. Unprepared women do not show a particularly heavy incidence
of minor psychosomatic symptoms (C) or of psychopathological
symptoms (E) such as manifest anxieties or fantasies specific to
pregnancy. The general impression given, however, is that anxieties
connected with pregnancy and childbirth are stronger among unprepared than among prepared women, who have means of dealing with
these anxieties, both in the form of information that they receive and
in the form of interpersonal support that they are afforded by the
social context of preparation. The overall pattern of the results
appears consistent if we simply assume that, for unprepared women,
existing anxieties are less readily admitted and recognized as such.

CORRELATIONS BETWEEN DIFFERENT AREAS OF
NEGATIVITY

Table 21 gives the intercorrelations between all the different areas of
the negativity grid, and the correlations of the areas with total I,
total II, and the grand total.

Let us first examine the correlations within the first part of the grid.
The correlations between the partial scores for the four areas that
comprise the first part of the grid are on the whole rather low. This
finding justifies after the event the distinction made between the areas
in the construction of the grid. It indicates that each of these areas
does represent a specific area of interest in the personal history of the
women concerned. In other words, the scoring system used has
essentially avoided the danger of scoring the same item a number of
times, under different headings. Thus each of the partial scores for the
different areas, which are added together to form total I, makes its
own particular contribution to this total.

153

TABLE 21 INTERCORRELATIONS BETWEEN AREAS OF NEGATIVITY, PARTIAL TOTALS, AND GRAND TOTAL

		A	B	C	D	Total I	A	B	C	D	E	F	G	H	Total II
B	PPM	+·05													
	U	(−·02)													
C	PPM	+·13	+·23												
	U	(−·20)	(+·35)												
D	PPM	+·21	+·28	+·45											
	U	(−·24)	(+·32)	(+·57)											
Total I	PPM	+·44	+·60	+·83	+·62										
	U	(+·09)	(+·67)	(+·86)	(+·63)										
A	PPM	+·06	−·08	+·07	+·10	+·05									
	U	(+·14)	(+·14)	(−·13)	(−·10)	(+·02)									
B	PPM	+·01	+·06	+·13	+·02	+·11	−·07								
	U	(+·11)	(+·04)	(+·02)	(−·18)	(+·04)	(−·11)								
C	PPM	−·15	+·10	0	−·01	−·01	−·13	+·06							
	U	(+·12)	(+·36)	(+·08)	(−·18)	(+·21)	(+·14)	(−·11)							
D	PPM	+·01	+·31	+·10	+·19	+·23	−·02	−·04	+·03						
	U	(−·08)	(+·30)	(+·19)	(+·27)	(+·30)	(−·05)	(+·38)	(+·17)						
E	PPM	+·15	+·28	0	+·11	+·17	−·01	+·23	+·23	+·14					
	U	(+·15)	(+·04)	(−·19)	(−·11)	(−·11)	(+·45)	(+·22)	(+·02)	(−·06)					
F	PPM	+·05	+·24	−·02	+·19	+·10	−·05	−·20	+·29	+·32	+·25				
	U	(−·07)	(+·31)	(−·06)	(−·06)	(+·04)	(+·24)	(−·26)	(+·12)	(−·21)	(+·28)				
G	PPM	+·17	+·13	+·11	+·19	+·20	+·10	+·06	−·23	−·03	+·11	+·10	+·28		
	U	(+·39)	(+·38)	(−·14)	(−·13)	(+·13)	(+·03)	(−·11)	(+·20)	(−·06)	(+·04)	(+·24)	(+·08)		
H	PPM	+·09	0	−·08	+·06	+·08	+·09	−·19	−·05	−·03	−·06	+·05	+·28	+·24	
	U	(+·20)	(−·07)	(−·03)	(−·02)	(+·04)	(+·02)	(−·16)	(−·33)	(+·06)	(+·21)	(−·08)	(+·08)	(+·28)	
Total II	PPM	+·11	+·35	+·11	+·26	+·28	+·15	+·24	+·34	+·43	+·74	+·50	+·43	+·24	
	U	(+·36)	(+·45)	(−·12)	(−·15)	(+·17)	(+·41)	(+·17)	(+·35)	(+·21)	(+·62)	(+·41)	(+·68)	(+·28)	
Grand total	PPM	+·39	+·60	+·70	+·60	+·90	+·12	+·17	+·11	+·37	+·45	+·30	+·36	+·17	+·65
	U	(+·26)	(+·75)	(+·61)	(+·41)	(+·86)	(+·22)	(+·12)	(+·34)	(+·34)	(+·22)	(+·24)	(+·44)	(+·17)	(+·64)

The two areas most closely related are areas C and D (disturbed family background and difficulties in social adjustment). This association is easily explained by a factor common to both interpersonal and social difficulties, in the widest sense, including family problems.

The correlations between the different areas tend to be higher for the unprepared than for the prepared women. We have already seen that the former tend to have higher global negativity scores than do the latter. These two observations are, of course, related in the sense that a higher negativity score is likely to be spread over the various areas.

It is interesting too that, for unprepared women, negativity in area A (pathology) has a low negative correlation with negativity in areas C and D; there is no such correlation for prepared women. Thus women who report serious pathological antecedents would tend also to admit fewer family and social difficulties, and vice versa. It is clearly impossible to tell whether this negative relationship reflects only attitudes assumed at the time of the interview, or whether it reflects genuine experiential variables, but it is certainly a problem specific to the unprepared women. We have noted elsewhere that negativity with respect to previous pathology tended to be lower among unprepared women than among prepared women, whereas, conversely, family troubles were more frequent among them. There does therefore seem to be, among unprepared women, a certain tendency for these two types of disability to be mutually exclusive, as their negative intercorrelation would indicate.

Let us now examine the correlations within the second part of the negativity grid. The same general observation may be made as for the first part, namely, that the correlations are on the whole rather low. It is interesting here to analyse the correlations in rather more detail. Areas A and B, which represent general pathology and gynaeco-obstetrical pathology during pregnancy respectively, have no marked relationship with the other areas of negativity during pregnancy. One exception to this is the appreciable positive correlation between general pathology and anxieties connected with pregnancy and childbirth among the unprepared women (0·45). It would therefore appear that anxiety symptoms, although of no greater frequency among unprepared women (*Table 20*), are more directly related in their case to the pathological events that may occur during pregnancy.

155

Nor are the psychosomatic symptoms specific to pregnancy (C) – vomiting, lumbar pains, insomnia, etc. – very closely related to the other aspects of negativity during pregnancy. Such relationships as do appear cannot be explained in any coherent manner. Doubtless the most interesting point to note is that somatic and psychosomatic pathological manifestations during pregnancy seem to be totally unrelated to one another, at least in so far as the dividing lines adopted in the grid are concerned.

On the other hand, some of the psychological symptoms concerned show a greater degree of mutual coherence. Let us, for example, consider the intercorrelations between areas D, E, and F, which cover, respectively, problems connected with womanhood and motherhood, psychopathological symptoms in the form of anxieties specific to pregnancy and childbirth, and personality or behaviour disturbances which reflect these anxieties in a more indirect way. We find a relatively clear relationship between personality and behaviour disturbances (F) and each of the other areas. In contrast, there is no relationship between problems of womanhood and motherhood (D) and the specific anxiety reactions of pregnancy (E). This last finding may appear somewhat surprising, but in our view it can, in fact, be largely interpreted in terms of the considerable difference in level between the two kinds of material. Whereas disturbances connected with womanhood and motherhood always express deep-lying problems, whose origin is to be found in the woman's personal history and especially in the stages of her sexual development in early childhood, anxieties connected with pregnancy and childbirth, whether these involve fantasies about the baby (fears of abnormality, etc.) or fear of confinement itself, appear relatively superficial and of little personal significance. On the other hand, when such anxieties develop on a very large scale, they may lead to disturbed psychological reactions to pregnancy, and thereby to behavioural disturbances (correlations between E and F of 0·25 for prepared women and 0·28 for unprepared women). Here we have a general rise in the level of control and in defences against anxiety, which leads to certain modes of external expression in behaviour.

The relations between problems connected with womanhood and motherhood on the one hand, and disturbances of behaviour on the other, are less easily unravelled. There is an inverse correlation between these two areas, for prepared and unprepared women, respectively, being positive for the former ($+0·32$) and negative for the latter

(− 0·21). In order to try to understand this rather complex relationship, let us take the case of women who tend to reject their pregnancy and the coming of the baby (which is recorded as a negativity item in area D). If these are prepared women, one might expect to find direct behavioural expression of the problems that this rejection involves. Quite often, for example, these women will show depressive symptoms during pregnancy (recorded under F); hence the positive correlation. Among unprepared women, on the contrary, the existence of such an attitude of rejection decreases the probability of the appearance of depressive symptoms. This fits in quite well with the whole psychological picture that is emerging of unprepared women, who tend to compensate for their deep-lying problems by strengthening their defences at the most superficial level of behaviour or immediate social adjustment. Correspondingly, when manifestations of this kind do appear in the behaviour of unprepared women (*Table 20* shows that they appear as frequently among them as among prepared women), it would seem that these women make even greater efforts, during interview, to conceal their basic underlying problems, especially those connected with womanhood and motherhood.

With regard to this very complex structure of relationships associated with negativity during pregnancy, the present account has been limited to underlining some relationships that appeared sufficiently clear to be understood without too much difficulty, or, on the other hand, appeared to indicate especially well the wide range of possible interactions between the various manifestations of negativity during pregnancy. It is clear that in a field in which causal relationships are so complex and so closely dependent upon individual dynamic factors, a statistical study can do no more than contribute a few suggestions, whose true significance must wait upon further confirmation and individual clinical studies.

It may, finally, be of interest to consider some of the correlations between areas of the two parts of the grid. It has already been noted that the correlation between the two partial totals is low. Negativity in the personal history and negativity during pregnancy are therefore largely independent of one another, although one might have expected negativity during pregnancy to be more closely determined by negativity in the previous personal history.

If we examine the correlations of each area of 'past' negativity (Negativity I) with the total for negativity during pregnancy (Negativity

II), we find that the womanhood area has the highest correlation both for prepared and unprepared women (0·35 and 0·45 respectively). This finding is in line with the general hypotheses of our research, according to which pregnancy is to be regarded as one particular critical stage in the entire evolutionary course of womanhood. Among prepared women, past problems concerning womanhood reveal themselves most directly during pregnancy by the appearance of psychological symptoms (D, E, F), and not by somatic or psychosomatic symptoms. As always, the picture is much less clearly patterned for unprepared women, since, among the latter, problems concerning womanhood in their past experience reveal themselves, as in the case of prepared women, by extending into pregnancy (D), and also in the form of behavioural disturbances (F), but not by any particularly marked development of the specific anxieties connected with pregnancy and childbirth (E); on the contrary, these problems seem to find current expression in the superficial psychosomatic symptoms of pregnancy (C), and also in interpersonal difficulties within the family (G). The other areas of past negativity do not seem to have any clear connexion with the various manifestations of negativity during pregnancy. The only thing worth noting is a correlation, among unprepared women, between previous pathology and total negativity during pregnancy, with particular reference to interpersonal problems within the family.

An examination of the correlations between the different partial negativity scores, by periods and by areas, thus indicates the following:

(i) On the whole, these correlations are low. This suggests that the three different totals (total I, total II, and grand total) do indeed, as was intended, represent composite global indices to which each of the different areas and periods makes its own specific contribution, and that there is relatively little overlap between these contributions.

(ii) Certain relationships, however, do appear within the total area of negativity covered by the grid, and suggest that the grid can, up to a point, be used to provide a more differentiated picture of the women examined, a picture that tends to reflect certain psychological patterns. These patterns emerge fairly clearly from a comparison of the prepared and the unprepared women. It should therefore be useful to go beyond the simple correlating of the global index with the confinement scores, and to examine the relations between certain aspects of negativity and confinement. This will be attempted in Chapter 8.

Before going on to study the correlations between negativity and confinement, however, we must first see how negativity, as it has here been defined, is associated with certain general variables in terms of which the sample of women in the present investigation can be characterized. The following variables were isolated for this purpose: age, duration of marriage, sociocultural level, economic level, whether the woman was or was not employed, whether she was or was not Jewish (it was thought that this might be related to increased negativity because of traumatic events associated with the war), the wealth of material in the interviews, whether or not the woman had established good relations with the psychologist in the course of the interviews, and finally, for prepared women, motives for choosing the PPM.

As far as age is concerned, there is a small correlation with total past negativity (0·27 for prepared women. but only 0·11, statistically insignificant, for unprepared women). Age is not related to negativity during pregnancy for prepared women, but shows quite a marked correlation for unprepared women (0·40). It has already been noted that negativity tends to be greater during pregnancy among unprepared women than among prepared women; furthermore, the two groups do not differ significantly in average age. There seems therefore to be a rather specific relationship between age and difficulties in pregnancy in the case of unprepared women.

There is no correlation between negativity and duration of marriage, sociocultural level, or economic level. Jewish women seem to show greater negativity in their past history, but only among the unprepared women, so that this does not appear to represent a general characteristic of all the Jewish women in the sample. Whether the women are employed or not is unrelated to negativity.

The correlation between the amount of material in the case-history and the total negativity score is 0·21 for prepared women and 0·68 for unprepared women. This raises a fundamental methodological problem in our experimental design. Negativity was assessed entirely

159

on the basis of the women's own accounts of their personal history and their problems. It might therefore be that the total negativity score is higher in proportion to the degree to which the women were willing to confide information about themselves in the course of the interviews. This is a particularly difficult problem in the case of women who have a low overall negativity score, based on meagre interview material. May it not be that their true negativity is much higher than their score implies, and that it is only their reticence or the poor contact they make that prevents them from revealing their real difficulties? The results indicate that the possible non-validity of the measures obtained is not very serious among the prepared women: the correlation of 0·21 between amount of material in the interviews and total negativity score shows that the chances of finding high negativity are indeed rather greater for interviews with plenty of material than for interviews with relatively meagre material, but the correlation between the two variables is quite low. This is not, however, the case for the unprepared women, among whom the correlation is quite high. It would therefore appear that included in the group of women who make use of the opportunity afforded by the interviews to discuss their problems are those who tend most frequently to have high overall negativity scores; conversely, low negativity scores are found mainly among women whose interview records are meagre. This confirms the impression that unprepared women are, on the whole, likely to be more inhibited and less 'genuine' in their relations with the members of the research team. This might also explain why results for the unprepared women are often more unexpected, less coherent, and more difficult to interpret than are results for the prepared women. Some of these results, indeed, may have been distorted at the source by a tendency to be selectively reticent about particular areas of information. Such results have, in fact, frequently been interpreted in this way in the preceding pages. They have to be considered along with the correlations obtained between the quality of the relations established between the women and the psychologists during the interviews, and the total negativity score (0·34 for prepared, 0·24 for unprepared women). Here again we find that there is a certain association, but this time it is for both groups of women. It therefore appears that it is not in respect of the quality of their relations with the psychologists that the two groups differ, but in their capacity for revealing their actual difficulties in the course of these relations. In other words, the unprepared women

160

have no greater tendency than the others to refuse to establish contact, but seem to be inhibited in the expression of their problems by more basic and probably unconscious defences. Whatever may be the significance of the correlations which have been discussed above, it must be noted that, especially among the prepared women, they are all relatively small, which suggests that, on the whole, the negativity scores are relatively independent of the interpersonal factors at work in the interview situation, and that they probably do reflect reasonably accurately the actual disabilities under which the women may be suffering.

SUMMARY

The global index of negativity has an approximately normal distribution for the whole sample of subjects, and gives good discrimination. The negative items are on average more numerous in the first part of the grid (negativity in the personal history) than in the second part (negativity during pregnancy). They are more numerous for the adult period than for adolescence, and more numerous for adolescence than for childhood. On the other hand, the negative items occur with approximately equal frequency during the two successive stages of pregnancy. It must be remembered that we have to do here with factors reported by the women themselves in the course of the interviews. Their relative frequency therefore depends on a number of considerations – their real existence, the probability of their being reported, and the structure of the grid itself, which tends to itemize factors to a greater or lesser extent according to the areas concerned.

An examination of the correlations indicates that negativity in the personal history is heavily weighted in the global score compared with negativity during pregnancy. On the psychometric level, therefore, we might be tempted to limit the collection of information to the former. At a clinical level, however, the latter appears to be indispensable. It provides material of a very different kind, as is indicated by the low correlation between negativity in the personal history and negativity during pregnancy.

Negativity is higher among unprepared women than among prepared women, especially in the area of 'family background' in the first part of the grid, and for the whole of negativity during pregnancy (second part). Further, if we examine the intercorrelations between the

161

various aspects of negativity, we find that the unprepared women yield more complex patterns of correlation, which are in general more difficult to interpret, than do the prepared women. This is probably due to the fact that one encounters more problems in the past histories and greater disabilities in the personalities of these unprepared women, which cause them to adopt a more defensive attitude during the interviews. Some of the factors involved in the self-selection of the two groups (prepared and unprepared) may also be involved here. These factors must be taken into account in interpreting the differences between the two groups in connexion with confinement and with the relations between negativity and confinement.

As a result of these analyses, the negativity grid appears to be a useful instrument, well fitted to the task of handling the data provided by the interviews. The summation of the various negativity factors yields a discriminative global index. Moreover, an examination of the intercorrelations of the various parts shows that, between areas and periods, these are quite low. This indicates that the various categories of information do not overlap to any great extent. Some relationships do, however, stand out sufficiently clearly for us to distinguish certain well-defined 'individual patterns' of negativity, which offer, to some extent, an approach to the patterns of personality themselves.

CHAPTER 8

Relations between Negativity and Confinement

NEGATIVITY RELATED TO CONFINEMENT

Chapter 6 was concerned with the different aspects of confinement, as represented by the measures used, and their interpretation. Chapter 7 dealt with the negative aspects of the personal history and of the pregnancy, as revealed in the interviews, and with the patterns of interrelations between these aspects. In these two chapters, two types of data were studied separately, those concerned with confinement and with negativity, respectively. The present chapter attempts to establish the relation between these two sets of data.

CORRELATION BETWEEN NEGATIVITY AND CONFINEMENT

According to the hypothesis underlying the research, we might expect the women with the greatest amount of disturbance in their personal histories to have the poorest confinements. This is a hypothesis that can readily be tested in the present experimental population. Let us define a good confinement as one with a score of 22 or less, and low negativity as corresponding to a score of 20 or less.[1] We thus have four possible combinations, represented by the following subgroups:

A – women with low negativity who have a good confinement
B – women with low negativity who have a poor confinement

[1] In both cases we are dealing with values which enable us to subdivide the 116 women concerned (90 prepared and 26 unprepared) into two approximately equal subgroups, thereby contrasting 'good' and 'poor' confinements, and 'low' and 'high' negativity. We decided to define 'good' confinement and 'low' negativity by means of a single line of demarcation applied to the entire group of 116 women, whether prepared or unprepared. It is thus possible in the following analyses to establish comparisons between prepared and unprepared women in respect of the quality of the confinement and the significance of negativity.

163

C – women with high negativity who have a good confinement

D – women with high negativity who have a poor confinement.

Cases that fall in subgroups A and D support the hypothesis, whereas cases occurring in subgroups B and C refute it. It would, of course, be unreasonable to expect that no cases would ever occur in subgroups B and C; the hypothesis can be taken as proved provided that these two categories occur significantly less frequently than do A and D. It is a question, therefore, of the distribution of these four combinations in our sample population.

Table 22a presents this distribution for the 90 women prepared by the PPM, and *Table 22b* does the same for the 26 unprepared women.

TABLE 22   RELATION BETWEEN NEGATIVITY AND CONFINEMENT

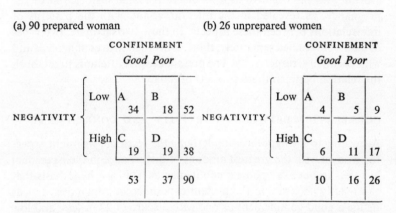

(a) 90 prepared woman

		CONFINEMENT		
		Good	*Poor*	
NEGATIVITY	Low	A 34	B 18	52
	High	C 19	D 19	38
		53	37	90

(b) 26 unprepared women

		CONFINEMENT		
		Good	*Poor*	
NEGATIVITY	Low	A 4	B 5	9
	High	C 6	D 11	17
		10	16	26

Of the 90 prepared women, 53 (59 per cent) fall in subgroups A and D, and the remaining 37 (41 per cent) in subgroups B and C; similar proportions (58 per cent and 42 per cent) are found among the 26 unprepared women. There is therefore a tendency in the direction of the predicted general relationship between negativity and confinement, but there are a great many exceptions. It is interesting, however, to examine the figures more closely. Among the prepared women, high negativity is accompanied by equal proportions of good and poor confinements (19 cases of each), whereas low negativity is associated with twice as many good confinements as poor ones (34 as against 18). Looking at the table the other way round, it appears that, when confinement is poor, high negativity is just as likely as low negativity (19 as against 18), whereas, when confinement is good, low negativity is twice as likely as high negativity. The interesting thing about *Table 22* is that it is asymmetrical and that the frequency of cases of prepared women showing low negativity and good confinement is particularly high (category A). Among the unprepared women, in contrast, the opposite combination (D) is the most frequent, that of high negativity with poor confinement. We shall return to this question when we examine the effects of preparation.

The finding that, when both prepared and unprepared women are considered, the association between negativity and confinement is not very close, is confirmed by the coefficient of correlation between the two variables. This is only 0·21 (significant at the 0·10 level) for the 90 prepared women and 0·19 for the unprepared women. These are very low correlations, and clearly show that the quality of an individual confinement cannot be predicted on the basis of negativity alone much beyond the level of random expectation. At the group level, however, there is some indication of a tendency towards the predicted relationship between high negativity and poor confinement, and between low negativity and good confinement. It may be recalled (cf. Chapter 5) that with a more restricted sample the pilot study found an appreciably higher correlation (0·46). We shall consider below some of the factors that may underlie this reduction in the size of the correlation.

FACTORS AND CONDITIONS IN THE EMERGENCE OF RELATIONS BETWEEN NEGATIVITY AND CONFINEMENT[1]

In the case of the pilot study, the correlation was calculated for a population consisting of both prepared and unprepared women. This in itself would mean that the correlation would be slightly higher. If, for the final sample, the calculation is made on the basis of all 116 women (90 prepared and 26 unprepared), we find that the correlation is 0·27 as compared with the correlations of 0·21 and 0·19 for the

---

[1] The matters that will be discussed below are supported by statistical analyses involving techniques which are too complex to allow of detailed exposition here (investigation of a large number of correlations between variables; assessment of partial correlations; components of selected and of matched subgroups, etc.). We shall here confine ourselves to summarizing the conclusions derived from these analyses.

two constituent samples. But this is not sufficient to explain the value of 0·46 found in the pilot study. If we make a closer examination of the data, we are led to the conclusion that three kinds of factor may contribute to the drop in correlation in the research proper:

(i) the characteristics of the sample population;
(ii) the characteristics of the measures used;
(iii) the nature of the facts studied, i.e. the psychological make-up of the women.

The characteristics of the sample population

Chapters 6 and 7, which dealt with confinement and negativity separately, showed that the scores for these variables tended to vary with the characteristics of the women concerned. In terms of the simple objective characteristics whereby the population was described, it appeared that negativity was on average higher among women who refused preparation, and perhaps also among older women; that unprepared Jewish women showed higher negativity in their personal histories, etc. But psychological characteristics were also relevant: the refusal or acceptance, or even the seeking, of preparation by the PPM was, quite obviously, associated in many cases with the woman's personality; and these characteristics of personality influence the responsiveness to the interviews, just as they undoubtedly have repercussions on the confinement itself.

Now, if all these factors can affect both the negativity score and the confinement score, it is reasonable to suppose that they can also affect the correlation between the two. It is likely that different correlations between negativity and confinement would be found for a group of intelligent and cultured women and for a group of women of low intellectual and cultural level; and that the correlations would differ according to whether the groups consisted of women of low or of high negativity, who accepted or refused preparation, etc. None of the obtained correlations would be any more 'accurate' that the others; each would reflect the relationship for the type of women considered. We had certainly attempted to secure an unselected group, but it must be remembered that factors of selection were involved in the study from the start. Indeed, although in the first instance all the women who met the basic criteria were included, complete records could be compiled for only 116 out of more than 200, for reasons already discussed in Chapter 4 – and these, of course, require to be taken into consideration.

Instead of looking for an illusory 'true' value for the correlation between negativity and confinement, it would appear more useful to try to explain the obtained values, i.e. 0·21 for the prepared women and 0·19 for the unprepared women, and to try to understand why the correlation is lower in the research sample than in the pilot study. An examination of the psychological characteristics of the women contributes to this end, as will presently be shown.

The characteristics of the measures used

No measure is perfect, and in the preceding chapters the possible disadvantages of the measures used in the present research have been fully discussed. In the present context, special attention should be paid to the possible effect on the correlation between negativity and confinement of the fact that some of the low negativity scores are probably ambiguous, as mentioned at the end of the previous chapter. Among women who get low negativity scores, the majority no doubt actually suffer from minor disturbances only; but in all probability there are also some instances where, in spite of very real disabilities, the women have not freely confided during the interviews and hence have received a low negativity rating. Clinically, such scores can be regarded as suspect, but when the correlation is calculated, the scores have to be used as they stand. Thus there may be women who have poor confinements because of serious pre-existing difficulties but who, on interview, have adopted a defensive attitude which leads to their being given a low score. In the statistical analysis, such cases appear to disprove the hypothesis of a correlation between poor confinement and high negativity. Even a relatively small proportion of such cases in the experimental population is sufficient to reduce considerably the size of the correlation.

If the 'meagre records' are suspect, then the correlation should rise when they are eliminated, and this is in fact what happens. If we exclude from the group of 90 women prepared by the PPM 27 records assessed as meagre, we find that the remaining 63 records provide a correlation between negativity and confinement of 0·26 (instead of 0·21 for the whole group). If we exclude from the group of 26 unprepared women the 6 meagre records, we find a correlation of 0·54 (instead of 0·19). We shall see later that, in this latter case, the meagreness or otherwise of the records is not the only factor involved. For both prepared and unprepared women, however, the elimination of the meagre records does actually produce the expected rise in the correlation.

The psychological make-up of the women

As has been shown above, if we retain only the more prolific records, we find a much higher correlation between negativity and confinement for unprepared women (0·54 for a sample of 20) than for prepared women (0·26 for a sample of 63). A correlation based on only 20 cases must certainly be regarded with caution. The question is whether its size is connected with the absence of preparation. If so, then we have to think of preparation as tending to destroy the causal connexion between negativity and confinement.

To throw light on this point, a group of 20 prepared women was selected, directly comparable with the group of 20 unprepared women for whom the correlation of 0·54 between negativity and confinement was obtained. These 20 women were selected from those with the fuller records, and were matched with the unprepared women for age and sociocultural level. The hypothesis suggested above was not confirmed. The correlation between negativity and confinement for these 20 prepared women was in fact 0·62, compared with the correlation of 0·54 for the 20 unprepared women. It cannot, therefore, be maintained that preparation in itself tends to destroy the relationship.

It does, nevertheless, appear that we have here two subgroups of women the study of whom is of particular interest for unravelling the possible relationship between negativity and confinement. What, then, are the characteristics of these women? If these can be established, we shall be in a better position to specify the necessary conditions required for a high correlation, or, in other words, the conditions under which the sum total of the difficulties comprised in negativity adversely affect the quality of the confinement. It is easy to show the main distinguishing characteristics of these women, simply by comparing them with the rest of the sample, for whom the correlation between negativity and confinement is much lower. This comparison cannot, of course, be made for the unprepared women considered separately, since the group for whom a high correlation was obtained (0·54) consists of 20 women and there are only 6 other subjects. But it can be made for the prepared women, since in this case there are 20 women in the group with a high correlation (0·62) and 70 others (correlation for all 90 women: 0·21).

For these two groups of prepared women, consisting of 20 and 70 cases respectively, the means of some 50 variables considered *a priori* to be of interest were calculated. These variables included those of a general order concerning the women, variables concerning negativity, and variables concerning confinement. *Table 23* gives the values obtained for 18 of these variables, for which there was a marked difference between the two groups. The 20 women in the first group had better confinements than did the other 70, and, in particular, their behavioural control was better; they were more active during their confinement, used the PPM techniques better, established better relations with the staff, and, finally, had a more positive initial relation to the child. Negativity during pregnancy was, however, higher in their case. This may doubtless be explained, at least in part, by the picture of these women that can be deduced from the 'general variables'. They were more dependent during the interviews, and proffered more information (more productive interviews). Their greater assiduity in preparation no doubt also reflected in some degree this desire for contact. In addition, they tended to marry younger and to come from a lower sociocultural and economic level.

We have thus a picture of a group of women who approach pregnancy, preparation, and confinement with an attitude of greater dependence on specialized help, and probably also with greater confidence. Being more assiduous in preparation, they expect more of the PPM techniques, and practise them more conscientiously. Those with low negativity succeed, thanks to these attitudes, in achieving a good confinement. Within this group, however, certain other women, with high negativity, approach pregnancy with misgiving, and react to its progress with a degree of anxiety which is reflected in high negativity during pregnancy. For them at least, dependence on the specialists and faith in the PPM afford reassurance against their anxiety. But this anxiety, which probably indicates a whole complex of problems in existence long before pregnancy, tends to lead to a poor confinement, and in these cases the PPM techniques are not sufficient to ward off the poor confinement. This would account for the direct link, among women of this type, between negativity and poor confinement. Married young, relatively uncultured, dependent, and endowing preparation with a kind of magical power to help them in

TABLE 23   MEANS, ON 18 VARIABLES, FOR TWO SUBGROUPS
OF PREPARED WOMEN

Variables	Means for 20 prepared women showing a high correlation (+·62) between negativity and confinement	Means for the 70 other prepared women	Interpretation of results in respect of the subgroup of 20 women
GENERAL VARIABLES:			
Years married	2·05	2·37	Married younger
Cultural level	1·40	2·70	Lower cultural level
Socio-economic level	9·75	11·47	Lower socio-economic level
Fullness of interviews	1·00	0·61	More complete interviews
Dependence shown during interviews	1·70	1·13	More dependent during interviews
Assiduity in preparation	0·15	0·30	More assiduous in preparation
CONFINEMENT:			
Pain	9·60	10·90	Lower pain score (less pain)
Behavioural control	9·35	11·06	Lower behavioural control score (better behaviour)
Total score (pain plus behaviour)	19·10	21·74	Lower total confinement score (better confinement)
Activity	1·55	1·89	More active
Relations with staff	0·70	1·13	Better relations with staff
Relation to baby	0·60	0·89	Better relation to baby
Breathing technique	0·75	1·07	Better breathing technique
Relaxation technique	1·05	1·47	Better relaxation technique
Bearing-down technique	0·75	1·00	Better bearing-down technique
NEGATIVITY:			
Negativity in personal history (I)	13·05	12·90	Same negativity in personal history
Negativity during pregnancy (II)	8·20	7·41	Higher negativity during pregnancy
Total (I + II)	21·25	20·21	Higher total negativity

the face of the threats of confinement, they are poorly equipped to defend themselves, during childbirth, against the flood of anxiety which it arouses. When the burden of anxiety is too heavy, reassurance is ineffective, the techniques learned are insufficient, and the confinement is poor.

Among the better equipped women (less recently married, higher sociocultural level, more reasoned views on the value and limitations of the PPM, less dependence on the specialists, etc.), one would, correspondingly, expect that the threat of potentially severe anxiety would be less directly expressed in poor confinement. Less vulnerable, owing to a less naïve faith in the PPM, to the uncertainties of the experience of confinement, they discover within themselves greater resources and means of defence against these hazards. In the more extreme cases, then, one would expect to find women with very high negativity who defend themselves sufficiently well against the threat of anxiety to prevent it from disorganizing the pattern of confinement, and who, in spite of their burden, have a good confinement. It might well be that there are enough cases of this kind among the 90 prepared women to cause the correlation between negativity and confinement to fall to the relatively low level of 0·21.

The emphasis is therefore on the relatively direct expression of negativity in poor confinement. The hypothesis positing a relationship requires to be reformulated: negativity is certainly *always* a possible factor in poor confinement, but it is an actual factor only under certain conditions, i.e. if the woman's personality allows this negativity to disorganize the controlled patterns of behaviour which are expected of her by the staff of the labour ward. This is, of course, only a hypothesis, but some additional arguments can be advanced in its support.

SOME ASPECTS OF GOOD CONFINEMENT RELATED TO
NEGATIVITY

The hypothesis of a relationship between negativity and confinement has been discussed in the preceding section. A study of the two populations involved (90 women prepared by the PPM and 26 unprepared women) shows that such a relationship exists, but that it applies only to a limited proportion of the subjects. Indeed, this is quite obvious from the analysis given at the beginning of the chapter.

171

Four possible combinations were there distinguished:

A – low negativity and good confinement
B – low negativity and poor confinement
C – high negativity and good confinement
D – high negativity and poor confinement.

It was thus shown that, with or without preparation, subgroups A and D (supporting a relationship between negativity and confinement) comprised approximately 60 per cent, and subgroups B and C only 40 per cent of the women. But we are left with the question of what distinguishes the women in subgroups A and D, whose results support the hypothesis, from those in subgroups B and C, whose results do not. Among the women with low negativity, for example, some have a good confinement and others have a poor confinement. One would like to know whether these two types of women show different characteristics which might be relevant to the difference in the quality of their confinements.

An attempt was made to locate such differences by calculating, for a whole series of variables, the means for each of the four subgroups A, B, C, and D. The variables included in this calculation were selected on the basis of the results and considerations discussed in the preceding section, and of a whole series of statistical analyses which cannot here be considered in any detail. *Table 24* gives the relevant means, and reveals a whole series of differences between women who have a good confinement and women who have a poor confinement. These differences, moreover, appear to form a coherent overall pattern.

DIFFERENCES OBSERVABLE DURING PREPARATION

Let us consider the *prepared* women with low negativity scores, and compare those who have a good confinement with those who have a poor confinement (subgroups A and B).

The women who have a good confinement have more productive interviews than those who have a poor confinement, despite the fact that they are of slightly lower sociocultural level. This is much more a reflection of their mode of contact (greater dependence during the interviews) than of the amount of negative material they have to disclose. Their negativity is, in fact, particularly low, especially in regard to problems connected with womanhood and with their past history. Here, therefore, we find evidence for the association between

172

TABLE ... MEANS, ON 15 VARIABLES, FOR SUBGROUPS CONSTITUTED IN TERMS OF NEGATIVITY AND CONFINEMENT

Negativity / Confinement	90 women	Prepared women				26 women	Unprepared women				High score indicates:
		A low good	B low poor	C high good	D high poor		A low good	B low poor	C high good	D high poor	
Sociocultural level	2·41	2·44	2·61	2·42	2·16	1·27	0·75	1·20	1·50	1·36	High sociocultural level
Fullness of interviews	0·70	0·68	0·50	0·89	0·74	0·80	0·75	0·20	1·00	1·00	Productive interviews
Dependence during interviews	1·25	1·15	0·88	1·63	1·42	1·34	1·50	1·20	1·00	1·54	Dependence during interviews
Motivation for PPM	0·76	0·65	0·84	0·53	1·05	—	—	—	—	—	No great motivation for PPM
Duration of confinement	8·82	8·59	8·44	8·32	10·11	7·61	7·25	6·20	7·33	8·54	Long confinement
Activity	1·81	1·53	2·22	1·47	2·16	1·80	1·50	2·00	1·16	2·36	Little activity during confinement
Relations with staff	1·03	0·68	1·44	0·68	1·37	1·46	1·00	2·20	0·16	2·00	Poor relations with staff
Relation to baby	0·82	0·62	1·44	0·53	1·00	1·30	1·50	1·40	0·66	1·54	Poor relation to baby
Breathing technique	1·00	0·44	1·72	0·79	1·58	—	—	—	—	—	Poor technique
Relaxation technique	1·38	0·85	2·22	1·05	1·58	—	—	—	—	—	Poor technique
Womanhood	4·18	3·03	4·50	4·79	5·79	3·96	2·00	1·40	3·83	5·90	Difficulties in relation to womanhood
Negativity in personal history	12·93	8·80	10·72	17·95	17·63	14·15	7·25	7·20	17·16	18·18	Appreciable negativity in personal history
Negativity during pregnancy	7·59	6·20	6·50	8·42	10·74	9·38	7·25	6·40	9·67	11·36	Appreciable negativity during pregnancy

negativity and confinement within the subgroup of women of low negativity: it is the women who have the best confinements who show the lowest negativity.

Similar relationships are to be found among women of high negativity (group C – good confinement, and group D – poor confinement): more productive interviews, greater dependence and desire for contact, and lower global negativity for good confinements than for poor confinements.

This attitude of dependence, of desire for contact and reassurance during the interviews, is associated, in the case of women who have a good confinement, with a particularly high level of motivation in relation to preparation, as is shown in *Table 25*. Motivation is strong

TABLE 25   MOTIVATION FOR PREPARATION IN FOUR SUBGROUPS
CONSTITUTED ACCORDING TO DEGREE OF NEGATIVITY AND
SUCCESS OF CONFINEMENT
($N = 90$)

		LOW NEGATIVITY		HIGH NEGATIVITY		
		A *Good*	B *Poor*	C *Good*	D *Poor*	
		Confinement		*Confinement*		
MOTIVATION FOR PPM	0 = strong	18	6	11	4	39
	1 = medium	10	7	6	10	33
	2 = weak	6	5	2	5	18
		34	18	19	19	90

in 43 per cent of the women (39 out of 90). It is strong rather more frequently when negativity is low (A and B combined, 24 women out of 52, or 46 per cent) than when it is high (C and D combined, 15 women out of 38, or 39 per cent). But the association is much clearer with the quality of the confinement than with negativity. In fact, for low negativity, strong motivation for the PPM appears in 53 per cent of the women who have a good confinement (A), but is much less frequent (33 per cent) among those who have a poor confinement (B).

In the case of high negativity, the corresponding figures are 58 per cent (C) and 21 per cent (D), showing an even more marked difference.

The correlation between motivation for the PPM and the success of the confinement is 0·58 for the 38 women with high negativity compared with only 0·31 for the 52 women with low negativity. It would therefore seem that, when the burden of difficulties which the woman has to carry is heavy, motivation for preparation is a particularly important factor in the success of the confinement, compensating for these difficulties. Thus women who are likely to have a good confinement are characterized, from the beginning of preparation, by a more receptive, dependent, and accepting attitude with respect to preparation; and the greater the weight of the burden indicated by high negativity, the more marked this tendency is.

DIFFERENCES OBSERVABLE DURING CONFINEMENT

At the time of the confinement itself, women who have a good confinement are more active, and the difference in this respect between women who have a good confinement and those who have a poor confinement is of the same order, whether negativity is high or low. Further, in good confinements, PPM techniques are used more effectively, as is shown by *Tables 24, 26,* and *27.*

Among women with low negativity, breathing techniques are appropriately used (score of zero) in 52 per cent of the cases (27 out of 52, subgroups A and B combined). They are used equally adequately by only 39 per cent of the women with high negativity (15 out of 38, subgroups C and D combined). The same is true of relaxation techniques (29 per cent as against 21 per cent). It therefore appears that high negativity constitutes in some degree an impediment to a good confinement in these technical aspects, and that it is one of the factors underlying failure when the total of pre-existing difficulties is particularly high. It is not, however, the only factor, for here again the difference is more marked as a function of the confinement itself than as a function of negativity. In fact, among women who have good confinements, 62 per cent practise the correct techniques of breathing (33 out of 53, subgroups A and C combined) and 38 per cent the correct techniques of relaxation (20 out of 53); whereas the corresponding proportions fall, respectively, to 24 per cent and 8 per cent among those who have poor confinements (subgroups B and D combined). The

TABLE 26 USE OF BREATHING TECHNIQUES IN FOUR SUBGROUPS
CONSTITUTED ACCORDING TO DEGREE OF NEGATIVITY AND
SUCCESS OF CONFINEMENT
(N = 90)

| | | LOW NEGATIVITY | | HIGH NEGATIVITY | | |
| | | A Good | B Poor | C Good | D Poor | |
		Confinement		Confinement		
	Good 0	23	4	10	5	42
USE OF BREATHING TECHNIQUES	1	9	5	6	11	31
	2	0	1	0	0	1
	Poor 3	2	8	3	3	16
		34	18	19	19	90

TABLE 27 USE OF RELAXATION TECHNIQUES IN FOUR SUBGROUPS
CONSTITUTED ACCORDING TO DEGREE OF NEGATIVITY AND
SUCCESS OF CONFINEMENT
(N = 90)

| | | LOW NEGATIVITY | | HIGH NEGATIVITY | | |
| | | A Good | B Poor | C Good | D Poor | |
		Confinement		Confinement		
	Good 0	15	0	5	3	23
USE OF RELAXATION TECHNIQUES	1	14	7	11	9	41
	2	0	0	0	0	0
	Poor 3	5	11	3	7	26
		34	18	19	19	90

difference in the proportions is especially marked when negativity is low (68 per cent as against 22 per cent for good use of breathing techniques, for good (A) and poor (B) confinements respectively, and 44 per cent as against zero for good use of relaxation techniques).

Adequate use of the techniques thus seems to represent a factor in the success of a confinement, which is more important in cases where negativity is low. Indeed, we find that the correlation between adequacy of breathing techniques and quality of confinement is 0·66 for women with low negativity and only 0·43 for women with high negativity. The correlation between adequacy of relaxation techniques and quality of confinement is similarly higher among women with low negativity (0·71) than among women with high negativity (0·43).

Thus, generally speaking, women who have good confinements are characterized by better use of PPM techniques and greater activity, supported by more positive motivation and better participation. As has been emphasized, this attitude can be observed from the start of preparation. All this was already suggested by the findings discussed in Chapter 6. But if we take into consideration the factor of negativity, further facts are introduced: among women of *high* negativity, motivation for the PPM is of greater consequence for the success of the confinement, whereas among women of *low* negativity, the practice of the techniques appears to be of greater import. We shall discuss the significance of these points later. In the meantime, we shall continue our analysis of the data and show that findings are similar with respect to relations with staff (*Table 28*) and relation to the baby (*Table 29*).

Relations with staff were recorded as good (score of zero) for 36 (or 40 per cent) of the 90 women, and these good relations were equally frequent for low negativity (subgroups A and B combined, 40 per cent) and for high negativity (subgroups C and D combined, 39 per cent). During the confinement itself, therefore, negativity is not a factor in poor relations with the staff. The results, of course, indicate only general tendencies. While it is quite likely that certain kinds of difficulties do in fact contribute to poor relations, others on the contrary contribute to what are here defined as 'good' relations, especially where the woman's problems induce her to seek help and reassurance from the staff in a particularly dependent and defenceless way. However that may be, *Table 28* clearly shows that good relations with the staff constitute a very definite aspect of good confinement. They appear, in this respect, in 55 per cent of the women who have good confinements (29

177

TABLE 28 RELATIONS WITH STAFF IN FOUR SUBGROUPS
CONSTITUTED ACCORDING TO DEGREE OF NEGATIVITY
AND SUCCESS OF CONFINEMENT
($N = 90$)

		LOW NEGATIVITY		HIGH NEGATIVITY		
		A	B	C	D	
		Good	Poor	Good	Poor	
		Confinement		Confinement		
	Good 0	19	2	10	5	36
	1	8	8	5	5	26
RELATIONS WITH STAFF	2	6	6	4	6	22
	Poor 3	1	2	0	3	6
		34	18	19	19	90

out of 53, subgroups A and C), but in only 19 per cent of those who have poor confinements (7 out of 38, subgroups B and D). Here again, the difference is more marked when negativity is low (56 per cent for A and 11 per cent for B) than when it is high (53 per cent for C and 26 per cent for D). This factor, therefore, has more influence upon the success of the confinement in women with *low* negativity (0·73) than in women with *high* negativity (0·43).

Among women who have good confinements, the relation to the baby, at the first contact after birth, is also far better. This observation, which probably provides one of the keys to the attitude of women who have good confinements, is illustrated by *Table 29*, which allows conclusions very similar to those discussed above. Here again, a good relation to the baby is more clearly a factor in good confinement among women of *low* negativity ($r = 0·57$) than among women of *high* negativity ($r = 0·33$).

We have, therefore, a fairly coherent picture of the women who have good confinements. During pregnancy, their more productive interviews indicate better contact with the hospital staff and more positive

TABLE 29 RELATION TO BABY IN FOUR SUBGROUPS
CONSTITUTED ACCORDING TO DEGREE OF NEGATIVITY
AND SUCCESS OF CONFINEMENT
(*N* = 90)

| | | LOW NEGATIVITY | | HIGH NEGATIVITY | | |
| | | A *Good* | B *Poor* | C *Good* | D *Poor* | |
		Confinement		*Confinement*		
RELATION TO BABY	Good 0	20	4	11	7	42
	1	8	7	6	7	28
	2	5	2	2	3	12
	Poor 3	1	5	0	2	8
		34	18	19	19	90

motivation for preparation. During confinement itself, these women have better relations with the staff of the labour ward, are more active, practise PPM techniques more efficiently, and, finally, show a better relation to the newborn baby. The opposite is the case for women who have poor confinements. These findings therefore essentially confirm the conclusions of Chapter 6.

One obtains the same contrasting pictures in the case of unprepared women, excluding of course the aspects ·relevant to preparation (motivation and practice of techniques), and the impressions are perhaps a little less clear, although we cannot say how far this is due to the absence of preparation, or to the small number of cases or factors of selection in the group.

These observations are valid for the women in general, but finer distinctions appear when negativity is taken into account. *Table 30*, which summarizes the findings referred to above, for the prepared women, shows this to be the case. Among women of *low* negativity, good confinement is *particularly* related to adequate use of the techniques, good relations with the staff, and a good relation to the

179

baby. Among women of *high* negativity, these factors are less significant; but, on the other hand, the initial motivation for the PPM is a
much more important determinant.

TABLE 30   CORRELATIONS BETWEEN QUALITY OF CONFINEMENT
AND 5 VARIABLES FOR TWO SUBGROUPS OF DIFFERENT NEGATIVITY

Correlations between quality of confinement and:	Women prepared by PPM		Total (*N* = 90)
	Low negativity (*N* = 52)	High negativity (*N* = 38)	
PPM motivation	+·31	+·58	+·31
Breathing technique	+·66	+·43	+·63
Relaxation technique	+·71	+·43	+·60
Relations with staff	+·73	+·43	+·45
Relation to baby	+·57	+·33	+·35

It thus seems that, when the burden of pre-existing difficulties is
heavy, the factors governing success are not so much a satisfactory
reaction to the experience of confinement, or appropriate use of the
techniques; rather is it those women who have been strongly motivated
initially towards preparation who will have good confinements (this
does not, of course, exclude other possible factors; it goes without
saying that it is an advantage if the techniques are properly applied
and if the psychological reaction to confinement is favourable). It may
well be that, for these women, strong motivation for preparation
reflects a very special need for reassurance, which is effective when it
is sufficiently genuine. Women with less severe difficulties (low negativity) rely to a lesser extent upon this initial commitment to preparation for the future success of their confinement, and among these
women the determinants of success are more objective (proper use of
the techniques) and more genuinely indicative of satisfactory psychological reactions to pregnancy and confinement (good relations with
the staff and good relation to the baby).

180

CONCLUSIONS

The negativity score includes, by its very nature, all those factors which, constituting and expressing the woman's total burden of problems, affect both pregnancy and confinement. It has been shown that the extent of this total burden of negativity does bear some relation to poor confinement, but that the relationship is not a very close one ($r = 0.21$ for 90 prepared women, and $r = 0.19$ for 26 unprepared women). The hypothesis was therefore advanced that other psychological factors might be associated with good and poor confinements, in particular, the *conditions* under which the psychological disability manifests itself in poor confinement. The results reported above elucidate some of these factors and conditions. They show, first of all, that the relationship between negativity and confinement is particularly close for the less robust, dependent women, who are poorly equipped to struggle with their personal problems on their own. We have seen, furthermore, that the women who have easier confinements tend to be those who approach pregnancy and childbirth with an attitude conducive to good contact and realistic demands, who are thus more genuinely motivated for preparation, and who, during confinement, practise the techniques more effectively, are more active, and establish better relations with the staff and eventually with their baby. All these factors are more marked when negativity is low, and in such cases there is a particularly high proportion of good confinements.

But the factors involved are also operative when negativity is high. Then, the initial motivation for the PPM far more often represents an attempt to find reassurance against anxiety. When such reassurance is possible, the confinement is appreciably improved by preparation, the effect of which, in a substantial number of cases, compensates for the disadvantage of high negativity. When reassurance is not effective, however, and the burden of difficulties is heavy, the confinement is poor. It would thus appear that the woman's psychological approach to her pregnancy is indeed to some extent determined by the problems of her past history, and that these therefore affect, indirectly, the quality of her pregnancy. But this effect is not inevitable. In some cases there is no doubt a direct causal relationship (serious difficulties, which lead to an unsatisfactory approach to pregnancy and later to a poor confinement); but in many others the pattern is much more complex (serious difficulties leading to an attempt to find

181

reassurance in preparation, in relations with the staff, and in meticullous use of the techniques, which in turn results in a good confinement; or, on the contrary, few personal difficulties, but a negative approach leading to a poor confinement, etc.).

A more detailed analysis of the various aspects of confinement, on the one hand, and of the different 'areas' of negativity, on the other, may enable us to give a more precise account of these relationships.

ANALYSIS OF RELATIONSHIPS BETWEEN NEGATIVITY AND CONFINEMENT

What has been said so far about the relationships between negativity and confinement has been in very general terms, and each of these two variables has been regarded as a whole. We can, however, proceed to a more detailed analysis of the various aspects and stages of confinement, and the different areas contributing to the global negativity score, respectively.

This analysis may be approached from two different but converging directions. Thus we may consider, on the one hand, which aspects and stages of confinement are most influenced by negativity; and, on the other, which areas of negativity have most effect on childbirth. We shall examine the correlations given in *Table 31* from both these points of view.

EFFECTS OF NEGATIVITY ON DIFFERENT ASPECTS OF CONFINEMENT

Among prepared women, the global negativity score is more closely related to pain (0·30) than to behavioural control, the latter correlation being negligible (0·12). The opposite is the case among unprepared women: the correlation with pain is negligible ($-0·03$) whereas that with behavioural control is appreciable (0·30). A particularly heavy burden of difficulties thus tends to express itself in disorganization of behaviour among unprepared women, and in pain among prepared women. It has previously been demonstrated that preparation is of benefit mainly with respect to behavioural control, actual pain – at least as measured here – being less affected. It can therefore readily be understood that negativity finds less direct expression in disorganization of behaviour when behavioural control is firmer (prepared women, $r = 0·12$) than when control is less effective (unprepared

TABLE 31 CORRELATIONS BETWEEN VARIOUS ASPECTS OF NEGATIVITY AND CONFINEMENT

		First stage			Second Stage			Whole confinement		
		Pain	Behaviour	Total	Pain	Behaviour	Total	Pain	Behaviour	Total
Negativity I	PPM	+·22	+·14	+·20	+·15	+·12	+·14	+·24	+·13	+·20
	U	(−·12)	(+·31)	(+·16)	(+·14)	(+·21)	(+·40)	(+·02)	(+·31)	(+·21)
Negativity II	PPM	+·16	+·03	+·09	+·24	+·06	+·17	+·29	+·05	+·15
	U	(−·13)	(+·17)	(+·06)	(−·04)	(+·05)	(+·12)	(−·10)	(+·13)	(+·04)
Total negativity	PPM	+·25	+·13	+·20	+·20	+·10	+·16	+·30	+·12	+·21
	U	(−·15)	(+·33)	(+·15)	(+·09)	(+·19)	(+·37)	(−·03)	(+·30)	(+·19)
Womanhood	PPM	+·28	+·30	+·32	+·10	+·28	+·23	+·27	+·31	+·33
	U	(+·05)	(+·41)	(+·30)	(+·17)	(+·35)	(+·41)	(+·14)	(+·45)	(+·36)

women, $r = 0.30$). But this takes no account of the relationships between negativity and pain. Thus among prepared women, despite their better behavioural control, high negativity is associated with a high pain score ($r = 0.30$), since, as has been seen, preparation tends to discourage behavioural manifestations.

As far as the unprepared women are concerned, there is no correlation between negativity and pain, but high negativity finds direct expression in disorganization of behaviour, which betrays the underlying anxieties.

Let us now examine separately the two main stages of confinement (dilatation-transition and expulsion-issue).

Among *prepared women*, negativity has more effect on pain than on behavioural control at both stages, and a little more effect during the first stage (correlations of total negativity score with pain 0·25, and with behavioural control 0·13, for the first period; 0·20 and 0·10 for the second period).

Among *unprepared women*, negativity has more effect on behavioural control than on pain at both stages, and markedly more effect during the first stage. For dilatation-transition, the correlation between negativity and behavioural control is 0·33, high negativity being associated with disorganization of behaviour (and, conversely, low negativity being associated with good behavioural control). At the same time, however, *high* negativity tends to be associated with *low* pain ($r = -0.15$). This is, of course, a very modest relationship, but it might indeed be that in certain cases, and in view of the method that we have adopted in recording our observations, marked disorganization of behaviour is associated with relatively low actual pain. This correlation between pain and global negativity clearly distinguishes between the unprepared women, for whom the correlation is negative (-0.15), and the prepared women, for whom it is positive ($+0.25$). The opposite direction of the correlations between negativity and pain (-0.15) and negativity and behavioural control ($+0.33$) for the unprepared women explains the low correlation between negativity and total confinement score (0·15) for the first stage; but the correlation between negativity and confinement is appreciably higher for the second stage (0·37).

To summarize, we may say that:

(i) negativity has more effect on pain in prepared women, and more effect on behavioural control in unprepared women;

(ii) these effects are more pronounced during dilatation-transition, especially in unprepared women;

(iii) if we consider the confinement as a whole, the correlation with negativity is of the same order in both of the main stages for prepared women, whereas it increases clearly from dilatation to expulsion in unprepared women.

The effects of negativity, considered globally, thus vary with the different stages and aspects of confinement, taking into account the presence or absence of preparation. The pattern of results is, however, complex and not easy to interpret.

EFFECTS ON CONFINEMENT OF DIFFERENT ASPECTS OF NEGATIVITY

More definite results appear when we examine the effects of the different aspects of negativity on confinement. *Table 31* shows that, among prepared women, negativity in the personal history and negativity during pregnancy affect the confinement as a whole about equally. Negativity in the personal history, however, influences the first stage of confinement rather more than does negativity during pregnancy (0·20 as against 0·09). Among unprepared women, on the other hand, it is during the second stage that negativity in the personal history is of greater consequence than is negativity during pregnancy (0·40 as against 0·12).

It is not without interest that it is negativity in the personal history, rather than negativity during pregnancy, that affects the confinement. The former, which comprises all the difficulties that can accumulate during the subject's life previous to confinement, gives a more accurate index of the 'fund of anxiety' of which the latter form of negativity is largely but the current reflection, and it is easy to see why it should have the greater significance for the confinement.

The available data were in fact analysed in considerably greater detail, all possible correlations between each stage and each aspect of confinement on the one hand, and each area, sub-area, and period of negativity on the other, being calculated. There is little point in entering here into any appreciable detail. We shall refer only to one aspect of negativity which gave particularly good correlations with confinement, namely problems of womanhood (last variable in *Table 31*).

185

Problems of this kind clearly affect confinement, correlating 0·33 with the whole confinement for prepared women and 0·36 for unprepared women. They are especially of consequence for behavioural control, at the two main stages, in both prepared and unprepared women. The correlation is particularly high for unprepared women, among whom severe problems connected with the acceptance of womanhood tend to find expression in marked disorganization of behaviour (0·45 for the whole confinement). This is the aspect of confinement which, in the absence of preparation, is the most vulnerable.

The 'womanhood' area actually gives higher correlations with confinement than does the global negativity score. From the point of view of pure 'psychometric prediction' of the quality of a confinement, it might appear advantageous to confine investigation to this area alone, since the higher the correlation, the better the prediction. For more clinically oriented use, however, we should not limit ourselves to data concerning womanhood. The results presented and discussed in this and the two preceding chapters show that we are dealing with extremely complex realities, where psychometric prediction – if we accept its approach – cannot be more than a fairly distant aim. Each case must be considered in the light of all the information available, in order to obtain a kind of preview of the way in which the difficulties with which the woman is afflicted are, or are not, likely to express themselves during confinement. This kind of foresight is, in any case, probably less valuable at the present stage of research than is an understanding of the different types of confinement.

From the point of view of clinical prognosis, the effects of preparation, taking into account the psychological disabilities to which the woman is subject, remain the major problem, and to this we shall devote our final section.

THE EFFECTS OF PREPARATION AS A FUNCTION OF NEGATIVITY

Table 22 gave the number of women in each of the four combinations when negativity was dichotomized into low and high, and confinements into good and poor, and revealed two facts which have already been considered above:

(i) prepared women have better confinements than do unprepared women, as is confirmed by *Table 32*;

(ii) prepared women show fewer severe disabilities (*Table 33*).

TABLE 32   DISTRIBUTION OF PREPARED
AND UNPREPARED WOMEN ACCORDING
TO QUALITY OF CONFINEMENT

| | Confinement | | |
	Good	Poor	Total
PPM	53	37	90
U	10	16	26
Total	63	53	116

TABLE 33   DISTRIBUTION OF PREPARED
AND UNPREPARED WOMEN ACCORDING
TO DEGREE OF NEGATIVITY

| | Negativity | | |
	Low	High	Total
PPM	52	38	90
U	9	17	26
Total	61	55	116

These general findings probably reflect, as we have seen, a difference between the samples composing the two groups (in part due to acceptance or refusal of preparation), and perhaps differences of attitude during the interviews (women who refuse preparation possibly showing a more defensive attitude).

Let us now consider separately the case of the women with high negativity. *Table 34* shows that, when negativity is high, among prepared women, good and poor confinements are equally frequent,

187

TABLE 34   DISTRIBUTION OF 55 WOMEN
WITH HIGH NEGATIVITY SCORES ACCORD-
ING TO QUALITY OF CONFINEMENT

| | Confinement | | |
	Good	Poor	Total
PPM	19	19	38
U	6	11	17
Total	25	30	55

whereas among unprepared women, poor confinements are twice as numerous as good ones.

Let us similarly consider those women with low negativity (*Table 35*). Here, good and poor confinements are equally frequent among

TABLE 35   DISTRIBUTION OF 61 WOMEN
WITH LOW NEGATIVITY SCORES ACCORD-
ING TO QUALITY OF CONFINEMENT

| | Confinement | | |
	Good	Poor	Total
PPM	34	18	52
U	4	5	9
Total	38	23	61

unprepared women, whereas good confinements are twice as numerous as poor ones among prepared women.

In both conditions (low negativity and high negativity), therefore, preparation eliminates about half of the poor confinements. For an unprepared woman, high negativity is a serious disadvantage: about two-thirds of such cases have poor confinements. Low negativity represents a distinct advantage when it is combined with preparation: two-thirds in this category have good confinements.

We may now ask whether preparation itself is more effective, and therefore more desirable, among women with high negativity or women with low negativity. The results presented suggest that preparation is equally effective in either case, since in both cases it eliminates about one-half of the poor confinements, a gain of 50 per cent. But this is based on a simple frequency count, and it may be desirable to have a more quantitative index of the improvement derived from preparation. *Table 36* gives the average confinement scores, at two levels of negativity, for prepared and unprepared women respectively.

TABLE 36 MEAN CONFINEMENT SCORES OF
PREPARED AND UNPREPARED WOMEN ACCORD-
ING TO DEGREE OF NEGATIVITY

| | *Negativity* | | |
	Low	*High*	*Difference*
PPM	19·58	22·22	2·64
U	20·75	27·94	7·19
Difference	1·17	5·72	

Prepared women with low negativity have the best confinements (a low confinement score indicating a good confinement). Unprepared women with low negativity come next; and it is worth emphasizing that they have rather better confinements than do prepared women with high negativity. Unprepared women with high negativity have the poorest confinements, and confinements in this group are appreciably poorer than in the other three groups. The differences shown in the table deserve some attention. They indicate that, when negativity is low, the difference in the quality of the confinement between prepared and unprepared women remains small (1·17 in favour of preparation). It is much more striking when negativity is high. In this case, unprepared women have especially poor confinements; but

189

the beneficial effect of preparation is very important (difference, 5·72) since, with preparation, confinements, in spite of the disadvantage of negativity, are likely to be almost as good as for unprepared women with low negativity (22·22 as against 20·75).

If we examine the table the other way round, we find that negativity affects the quality of the confinement much more clearly among unprepared (7·19) than among prepared (2·64) women.

The asymmetrical nature of *Table 36* indicates, therefore, how much benefit can be expected from preparation according to the weight of the burden that the woman has to carry. When this burden is heavy, a poor confinement is very likely, but preparation enables this probability to be appreciably reduced. When the difficulties comprising negativity are relatively light, the confinement is likely to be good, even without preparation, and the latter, when it is given, provides only moderate additional advantages. We must, of course, remember that this discussion is based on mean values, and that there are many individual exceptions and variations. There are, for example, cases where the burden is so heavy and of such a nature that preparation has no effect, and the confinement is scarcely, if at all, improved; and cases of the opposite kind, where preparation appreciably improves a confinement which, in spite of low negativity, would probably have been a poor one without preparation. Despite such exceptions, preparation would appear to be an especially effective technique in counteracting the untoward effects on childbirth of particularly severe disabilities.

SUMMARY

When the women are divided into subgroups, separating those with good from those with poor confinements, and those with high from those with low negativity, we find that the women who have the best confinements more frequently have low negativity, and that, conversely, those who have poor confinements more frequently show high negativity. This suggests a correlation between negativity and confinement. When this correlation is calculated, however, it turns out to be quite low (0·21 for prepared women and 0·19 for unprepared women). Since the pilot survey, using a sample of 60 cases, had given an appreciably higher correlation, this discrepancy constitutes a problem for which an explanation must be sought.

It must first of all be emphasized that the value of the correlation necessarily depends upon the constitution of the groups studied, since this may involve factors likely to affect both negativity and confinement. The problem therefore is one of comparing subgroups of different kinds and of examining the variations in the resulting correlations between negativity and confinement for these subgroups. Conversely, and perhaps more interestingly, we may study those subgroups that yield a relatively high correlation, with a view to unravelling the characteristics and factors responsible for this high correlation. This procedure was in fact adopted, and a group of 20 prepared women was selected for whom the correlation between negativity and confinement was 0·62. Compared with the other 70 prepared women, these 20 women married younger, were of lower sociocultural level, were more conscientious in preparation, and provided more information during interview. On the whole, therefore, they gave the impression of being more immature and dependent, and to a greater extent than the others seemed to be seeking in preparation a kind of 'magical' reassurance. They also, on the whole, had better confinements (in particular, showing better behavioural control), were more active, made better use of PPM techniques, and established better relations with the staff and a better relation to their baby. When the burden of negativity among these women was too great, however, this kind of reassurance was not sufficient to provide adequate defences against anxiety and thus could not ensure the success of the confinement, which tended on the contrary to be particularly poor. This would explain the relatively high correlation between negativity and confinement for this group (0·62).

These conclusions are confirmed by the results of another kind of analysis, which endeavoured systematically to identify the factors involved in good confinement, taking into account negativity. When negativity is high, the most important of the factors associated with good confinement is motivation for the PPM. When negativity is low, it is the more 'practical' factors that are influential – use of PPM techniques, relations with the staff, and relation to the baby.

Within the general variable of negativity, negativity in the personal history seems to be of more significance for confinement than does negativity during pregnancy, though the patterns of correlations are complex, and can be appreciably altered by preparation. Attention

191

should, however, be drawn to the special relevance of problems concerning womanhood as possible sources of difficulty during pregnancy and confinement.

It is somewhat difficult to assess the effects of preparation on the basis of these data, particularly because of the problems of sampling discussed in preceding chapters. It is undeniable that preparation is likely to improve the quality of the confinement, but the improvement due to preparation is particularly marked among women of high negativity. Because of preparation, these women are able to achieve confinements comparable in quality with those of unprepared women of low negativity. The improvement effected by preparation is quite substantial since, in the absence of preparation, the confinements of women of high negativity are likely to be particularly poor. An improvement is also evident for women of low negativity, but in this case it is much less marked.

It therefore appears that if negativity is taken into consideration the effects of the PPM can be more accurately assessed. This is of very special interest in predicting the success of prepared childbirth.

CHAPTER 9

Conclusions

Both the impetus for the team research described in the present work, and its subject-matter, were very largely derived from the manifold problems which have most fortunately gained prominence through the increasingly widespread use of methods of prepared childbirth. The theoretical bases of these methods have not yet been sufficiently elucidated, and there still remain lively controversies among experts, as was made clear in Chapter 1. When the method proves effective, and pain is more or less completely allayed, what are in fact the means by which these results are attained? It is not sufficient merely to take note of the results, for these must also be explained; and the explanation of the mode of action of painless childbirth presupposes an understanding of the pain mechanisms obtaining during childbirth itself. At the first and most generally applicable level of explanation, the problem of analgesia and that of pain are thus so closely related that it is impossible to consider the former without reference to the latter.

But we are thus necessarily led to investigate these problems on a second – no longer general, but specific – level, viz., how is it possible to explain the variation in effectiveness of the methods of prepared childbirth in different women, from complete success to obvious failure? And indeed, at this second level, we are again faced with the complementary nature of the respective factors determining pain and analgesia. One might well ask why, even without preparation, there is still so great an individual difference in the degree of pain experienced during childbirth.

The fundamental problem, therefore, is that of pain in childbirth, and its psychological determinants. The research reported in the present work has been centred upon this theme. Needless to say, pain is not a simple entity, a clearly defined psychological phenomenon with definite physiological determinants. This is obvious as soon as one attempts to assess it in an objective manner. If we take the case of someone in pain, his behaviour, complaints, agitation, and appeals for help will all suggest a state of intense suffering. But another person who, in a similar situation, shows less obvious symptoms, will not thereby necessarily appear to suffer less: we might even conclude that he may in fact be experiencing just as much, if not indeed even greater, pain, but that he exercises better control over its manifestations.

This raises the question whether such control is likely to lessen the pain experienced, or to increase it, or to have no effect one way or the other; and also, why one person may exercise such a high degree of control, and another so little, over the external manifestations of pain. It appears that many factors are involved in these differences, and all of them point to the need for research in the area of personality studies.

Any research into psychological methods of analgesia during parturition is therefore inevitably focused on the problem of pain, and thereby must also necessarily lead to the investigation of the role of personality factors in childbirth. The present research was designed to meet these requirements. The concept may indeed appear ambitious, and the results less than might have been hoped for. Some appreciable contribution may, however, have been made to the formulation of problems and to the development of methods appropriate to their solution, as we shall attempt to demonstrate in summarizing the main points of our research.

One cannot embark on such a project without some theoretical perspective, and consequently, some working hypotheses. The theoretical perspective adopted was that of psychoanalysis, and in Chapter 2 we tried to show that such an approach is potentially fruitful. Psychoanalysis appeared to offer the best theoretical framework for our study at its true level – that of a study of personality, with all its experiential determinants and individual particulars, relating to the critical situation presented by pregnancy and childbirth. Such a crisis is, of course, in itself significant, but it can properly be understood only against the background of the woman's personal development. This is what we attempted to demonstrate in Chapter 3, on the basis of a critical review of the main aspects of the relevant literature. It therefore appeared that a study of pain in childbirth involved an investigation of the significance that each woman attaches to her first pregnancy and confinement, as events of major importance in her feminine role. It was decided that it would be necessary (a) to collect as much information as possible about the woman concerned, by means of the case-history as well as clinical observation; and (b) to subject the confinement itself to detailed psychological observation. In the latter procedure it is necessary to distinguish as clearly as possible between the behavioural manifestations of pain and the pain that is actually experienced. Here, particular emphasis must be placed on some highly significant types of behaviour and modes of experience – activity, relations with the staff of the labour ward, and first relation to the baby.

What has been said so far merely implies the selection of certain possibilities within a general theoretical framework. These have been detailed in Chapters 4 and 5, first, through the definition of the research population, and, second, through the presentation and discussion of the methods of research. Since it was necessary to select certain alternatives, others obviously had to be discarded. In any research, some such sacrifice is required when one proceeds from the level of general hypotheses to that of assembling and analysing the data. It is not possible here to discuss in detail the advisability of our selection of data; the reader should refer to Chapters 3, 4, and 5.

Two hundred primiparous women, attending a maternity department in a Paris hospital, were studied during their pregnancy and observed during their confinements. Some of them were prepared by the psychoprophylactic method, and others did not undergo preparation. Three semi-directive interviews conducted during pregnancy provided life-history and clinical data, and each confinement was observed by a psychiatrist who was present in the labour ward. His observations were supplemented by an interview that took place two or three days after the confinement, as also by purely obstetrical data. From a total of 200 women, 116 were selected for the final analysis, according to specific criteria. This analysis employed several methods of classification specially devised for the purposes of the research, the two principal procedures being the 'negativity grid' and the 'confinement scoring grid'.

The negativity grid summarizes, classifies, and quantifies the data provided by the interviews. It exemplifies in two ways the need for making choices from various possibilities, to which we have referred above. First, psychometrically, it was decided that, in order to facilitate statistical analysis, all available information should be reduced to simple frequencies in the 'cells' of the grid, and the loss of material

195

inherent in this kind of procedure was accepted. Second, in order that entries could be summed for different dimensions, it was necessary to have a single principal criterion for the selection of the items of information to be included, and it was agreed that only items indicating 'negativity' should be included – various traumatic and pathological occurrences, unfavourable events and circumstances, etc., which, generally speaking, might be regarded as constituting a burden of disadvantages likely, according to the hypotheses of the research, to have some effects on pregnancy and confinement. The items of information retained were then classified by areas and by periods.

The confinement scoring grid was intended to play the same part of condensing, classifying, and quantifying data. It provided for the recording, at four successive stages of confinement, of the quality of behavioural control and, more subjectively, of pain experienced. Here, again, various ways of adding partial scores were possible, the most inclusive providing a total score indicating the 'quality' of the confinement considered as a whole. In addition, various aspects were scored separately, namely the activity of the parturient woman, the use of PPM techniques, relations with the staff, and first relation to the baby.

Chapters 6 and 7 are focused on these two grids respectively, and attempt to achieve two aims:

(a) to examine the internal structure of each grid; in particular, a study of the ways in which the various scores are distributed and of the correlations between the partial scores and the total score shows that these are psychometrically valid methods, and that the threefold aim of condensing, classifying, and quantifying has been satisfactorily achieved;

(b) to demonstrate certain important findings resulting mainly from a systematic comparison of women prepared by the PPM with unprepared women; it is shown, as might have been expected, that prepared women have better confinements, and that their advantage is greater in respect of behavioural control than in respect of pain itself. The 'index of control' (which is reflected by the difference between the pain and the behavioural control scores) is significantly higher for the prepared women than for the unprepared; this advantage is more marked during dilatation-transition than during expulsion-issue. Furthermore, relations with the staff of the labour ward and the first relation to the baby are significantly better for prepared women.

The question arises whether advantage in these respects is really due to the PPM. A study of the negativity scores suggests that factors of sampling, of 'self-selection', are involved in the two respective groups (prepared and unprepared). Preparation was offered to all the women, and only a minority refused. It is reasonable to suppose that, in the sociocultural climate of today, refusal or acceptance of preparation depends upon motivational and psychological factors which might themselves be expected to affect pregnancy and childbirth. In fact, negativity is significantly higher, on average, among unprepared women: the family background of these women appears to be characterized more frequently by incidents and experiences of potentially 'negative' significance; and 'negativity during pregnancy' is higher as well. They therefore seem to be women whose past history and personality tend more frequently to include unfavourable aspects, and this in turn leads them to refuse preparation.

The two groups are therefore, to start with, not strictly comparable psychologically. Accordingly, it might appear impossible to decide whether the more successful confinements of the prepared women are due to preparation itself, to personality factors which would probably have led to a better confinement even without preparation, or (as seems most likely) to a combination of both these factors (Chapter 8). Several points must be borne in mind here.

In the first place, this kind of difficulty is inherent in most medical research aimed at assessing the effects of some kind of treatment, as soon as there is sufficient confidence in the treatment for it to be prescribed for all apparently suitable cases. The only way to obtain two strictly comparable experimental groups would be to prepare one-half of the women, selected at random (e.g. every second woman in the order in which they appeared for consultation), and not to prepare the other half, while also matching the two groups for certain general variables. This, however, would appear to be impracticable. It would be possible, even though the two groups were still self-selected (thus respecting the right of the patient to make her own choice), to retain only subgroups matched on various general characteristics and on certain personality tests. But 'matching' of this kind would in fact be more apparent than real, since the basic problem

197

remains: women accept or refuse preparation for reasons which are probably relevant to their confinements, and it would be extremely difficult if not impossible to match accurately in respect of the factors concerned.

Second, detailed statistical analysis reveals different patterns of relationship between the various items for prepared and unprepared women. In general, these patterns of relationship are simpler and easier to understand for prepared women. Some attempt can therefore be made to ascertain how far the better confinements of the prepared women are due to personality factors, to preparation, and to the interaction of preparation and personality.

Third, the various patterns of relationship are illuminated further by a study of selected subgroups. Thus, findings in respect of a subgroup of 20 prepared women, for whom the correlation between negativity and confinement was high (0·62), made it clear that there are certain *conditions* under which the causal link between the two variables is manifested. High negativity appears to be particularly likely to disturb the confinement when the woman is immature and dependent, and inclined to seek in preparation a kind of 'magical' reassurance against anxiety. When negativity is low, on the other hand, similar attitudes on the part of the woman can lead to a successful outcome, and a good confinement.

Fourth, the unfavourable effects of high negativity on confinement vary greatly in degree according to whether the woman is or is not prepared: they are much reduced among prepared women. Here it would indeed seem that the beneficial influence can really be attributed to preparation.

Finally, clinical data appear to indicate the importance of preparation. From the clinical point of view, it would appear that, if account is taken of the factors comprised in the negativity index, prognosis can be appreciably improved by making allowance for the psychological context within which preparation will have to operate. There is some quantitative evidence to support this view. Thus, an analysis of the factors involved in 'good confinements' indicates that, when negativity is high, it is the motivation to accept preparation that appears to be the essential determinant of the quality of the confinement. This suggests the idea that these women may be seeking reassurance in preparation. When negativity is low, more 'pragmatic' aspects are involved, such as use of PPM techniques, relations with the staff, and relation to the baby.

It therefore appears that, although the methodological objection to the non-comparability of the respective groups of prepared and unprepared women may seem a serious one, it is of far less significance if one takes into account the variety of analyses made possible by our methods of research. This is, indeed, by no means the least of the advantages offered by these methods.

The present research represents little more than a first approach, the aim of which is to define problems, hypotheses, and methods. It is hoped that, despite the hazards, uncertainties, and errors inevitable in an attempt to achieve an overall view of such complex problems, the research may have contributed something of value to future research in the field, which is so urgently needed.

From a practical point of view, the interview guides and the negativity grid, together with the confinement grid, may be of use to the clinician who wishes to improve his methods of observation. In this way, they may lead to the refining and perfecting of methods of preparation, the value and advantages of which would appear today to be beyond dispute.

It is admittedly almost impossible to measure pain; consequently, the figures given for analgesia obtained by different procedures have no absolute value. They do, however, express at least part of the truth. Analgesia by psychological methods is an unquestionable reality. Despite the difficulty of actually measuring analgesia in different individuals, it can be asserted that for many women the psychotherapeutic support provided undoubtedly contributes to the positive results obtained.

Apart from analgesia, an attempt has been made to demonstrate statistically some of the medical and obstetrical advantages of these methods: e.g. the beneficial effect on the pathological aspects of pregnancy; a reduction in the length of labour; the decreased incidence of complications during confinement; the smaller number of surgical (obstetrical) operations; the favourable influence on the puerperium (lactation, general hygiene, etc.); and the decreased incidence of resuscitation of the newborn infant. Some of these results, such as those influencing the pathology of pregnancy, are attributed by several authors to the psychosomatic effects of these methods; others, such as the lower incidence of resuscitation, are ascribed to the absence of excessive medication; and others yet, such as the reduction in the length of labour, are assigned to the combined action of these two factors.

Statistics of this kind are not entirely accepted by all obstetricians, and doubtless further evidence is needed to support them. It is, however, true that excessive medication is unquestionably harmful and that psychotherapy can hardly fail to pay dividends, in a general way, through beneficial psychosomatic effects. There are, however, other advantages that are not at present the object of quantitative assessment, but are none the less important for that. The use of the methods provides the women with a rewarding experience, since they express their satisfaction and most of them wish for further preparation in the event of another pregnancy. Inasmuch as childbirth is a primordial emotional experience for a woman, the fact that she experiences it in full consciousness and without undue suffering cannot but have favourable psychological consequences for the mother herself and for the establishment of the mother-child relationship.

There may perhaps be sceptics who feel that none of these results has been established beyond dispute. To these it might be answered that if, in the last resort, the methods achieved no more, the fact that they require, on the part of the physician and the hospital staff, an attitude towards the woman compounded of benevolence, emotional warmth, and humanity, would in itself represent a positive contribution to the progress of obstetrics; it would in large measure justify a high degree of interest in the methods of preparation and a desire that they should become the object of more extensive research.

APPENDIX I

Three Case-histories

First Case-history

This case was selected from our file of complete records because it is representative of the sample as a whole. It is neither particularly interesting nor unusual, and it is not a pathological history. Moreover, it was not selected in order to demonstrate the merit of the research hypotheses, but to illustrate two features of the present study:

(i) the semi-directive method used in the three interviews, and described in Chapter 4;
(ii) the kind of clinical material that came up during these interviews, and the way in which it developed as pregnancy proceeded.

The negativity grid (described and explained in Chapter 5) records and sums potentially pathogenic items connected with the woman's past history, particularly those concerning womanhood and pregnancy.

Observation of the confinement takes the form of notes made on the spot and aims at describing the essential aspects of the situation and the way in which these developed. Although it was not our intention to provide an elaborate account, these observations were oriented by, and based upon, the results of the methodological analysis given in Chapters 3 and 4. They are supplemented by an obstetrical and behavioural record provided by the midwives.

The confinement grid (described and explained in Chapter 5) records the significant facts and evaluates them by stages and globally. These confinement scores, in conjunction with the negativity scores, make possible a synthetic appraisal of the case, which will be found at the end of the case-history.

MRS N

FIRST INTERVIEW WHEN 2½ MONTHS PREGNANT

Mrs N is a young woman of 18 years of age, who immediately established good contact. She is fair, plump, and tastefully dressed – obviously well to do. Despite her youth, she has an attractive natural poise.

201

Information on civil status was asked for immediately (age, address, type of accommodation). Mrs N had been a secretary but had given up work on getting married. Her husband is a technician who is currently in the army. She went to live with her parents when her husband joined the army. 'I prefer to live with my parents since my husband is away,' she explained. 'That way I don't have to pay for lodgings, and life is easier.'

Choice of hospital. Mrs N had decided to attend clinics and to have her baby at the Hôpital Rothschild, partly because her sister-in-law had had a baby there and had been very satisfied, and partly because she knew that women were prepared there for childbirth and she has strong views about this:

> 'I've already read a book about preparation for childbirth . . . I thought it might reassure me to read about it . . . I have confidence in this method. [*Q.*][1] I'm not afraid of having a baby, but I like to know what's going on inside me. That's why I read books about pregnancy and childbirth. [*Q.*] I wanted in any case to know how it works, so I've already been trying the breathing techniques described in the book – just for practice.'

Desire to be pregnant. Mrs N explained that she had been married for more than a year and that, in fact, during the first year of their marriage she and her husband had agreed to avoid impregnation, by using the so-called temperature method. This year, the couple were both extremely keen on having a baby, and conception occurred through choice. She explained that the temperature method that they had chosen had been perfectly satisfactory, and that they had both refused to use mechanical methods of contraception because 'it's not natural and it spoils the pleasure . . .'; also that they liked to feel that they had some 'strength of character and willpower' by observing some degree of abstinence.

Menstrual cycle. Mrs N normally has a regular cycle of thirty-five days. The menstrual flow usually lasts five days and is not very copious. She has never suffered from dysmenorrhoea.

Present position of couple. The husband is due to be released from military service in three months. The couple have in fact been separated for four months from the time when he was sent to Algeria. Mrs N had gone to join her husband in North Africa, and had passed the first month of her pregnancy near him. When her periods stopped, she 'knew' at once that she was pregnant.

Symptoms. Mrs N did not claim to have suffered from any marked discomfort. She mentioned only a lessening of appetite and some aversions during

---

[1] [*Q.*] indicates a question by the interviewer.

the second month of her pregnancy. She attributed these to the unhygienic conditions in which she had been living in North Africa: 'The boy who prepared the food cut the meat with a dirty knife – that sickened me. It has left me with a dislike for meat. Now, I even hesitate to eat a steak.' She reported having vomited on one occasion only, and having had a few attacks of nausea provoked by her aversions to food.

From the beginning of the second month, she suffered from hypersomnia and sometimes disturbed sleep. When asked about dreams, she reported the following: 'I dreamed that somebody was strangling me.' And on further questioning: 'It was my husband.' Mrs N associated this dream with the rather traumatic experience of living in North Africa with her husband, which had involved a certain amount of danger. She used to stay all day in her room waiting for her husband to return.

In summary, she did not feel physically or psychologically in any way different, as compared with her condition before her pregnancy.

Family history. Her *mother* is 60 years of age, and in good health; she has had eight children. Mrs N described her mother as an active woman, quite intelligent, and very highly strung:

'I admire her a lot. She is a wonderful mother. She really brought us up very well. She is quite good-looking. Having children rather spoiled her looks – I mean, she's rather stout, but she's still a good-looking woman. She's always working about the house, she's always doing something. It was quite remarkable the way she brought us up, with plenty of affection. It must have been a bit of a strain for her, for it's no fun to bring up eight children, but I've a great admiration for my mother.'

She again described her mother as an anxious woman, emotional, sensitive, and devoted to her children.

She was questioned about her return to her parents' house as a married woman:

'It's a funny thing – I'm even closer to my mother . . . I got the impression that her relations with me were a bit different; in one way I was still her little girl, but there was all the same a kind of difference, it wasn't quite the same. In our relations, you might say that she took more notice of me because I was married and was expecting a baby. This was very nice for me, because it's the only time in my life that I've felt any real intimacy with my mother. Even so, my mother is rather reserved and rigid. She never told me about anything, when my periods started or when I was married. She never taught us anything about this kind of thing, and now, since I got married, her attitude to me is quite different. I had the feeling of speaking to a different woman. It was much nicer, I had gone up a step. I was no longer a little girl. [*Q.*] Yes, my mother is very prudish. She closes her eyes to things. She never told me about anything. For example, when my periods started, she never said a word about it.'

First menstruation. This was at the age of 13 years. Mrs N appears not to have found her first menstruation traumatic because she had been warned in advance by her sister and her sisters-in-law. She said that when she was quite a little girl she had already heard of it and had gone to her sisters-in-law for information. She would never have dared to ask her mother, and anyway she did not think her mother would have told her. When her first period came, it was she herself who went to buy sanitary towels, and her mother said absolutely nothing. When she was asked what she thought of this, Mrs N said:

'Of course I don't think it's right. I don't blame my mother, because that's the way she is. Perhaps it's got to do with her temperament; besides, the older generations were less open than ours; but I think you ought to tell children about it. Perhaps it would depend on the children, since it might shock them. [*Q*]. Yes, I say that because I remember one of my nephews who was disgusted at his mother because he asked her how babies came and she told him. She must have explained it too crudely, because for a week he wouldn't kiss her. I think he was really disgusted. I think you have to do that kind of thing very tactfully. It may be difficult, but that's no reason for not talking about it at all.'

Upbringing. Mrs N thus revealed a rather strict upbringing before her marriage. Her mother did not let her go out: 'I didn't really feel strongly that I wanted to. I think what's wrong with young people today is that they are allowed to go out far too soon, and they end up by not being able to enjoy things when the time comes.'

It is, however, noteworthy that Mrs N had met her husband and got engaged at 17, and was married at $17\frac{1}{2}$. Her husband was in fact her first boy friend, and had been a childhood friend, being the brother of one of her sisters-in-law. But they had lost touch and had met again when he was 20 years old. She explained with a smile: 'Perhaps that's why we fell in love. After we met, he very soon fell in love with me and talked of getting married.'

Mrs N has an elder sister who got married at the age of 26 after a very long engagement. Her husband was a foreigner, a Russian, and the girl's parents were rather opposed to the marriage on the grounds of wartime difficulties. In addition, Mrs N's mother was distressed at the prospect of the marriage, because she knew that her daughter would be going to America. Eventually, they got married: 'My mother accepted it because she is an intelligent woman. She realized that my sister's happiness was involved, and so she came round to accept it.'

204

Father. Her father is 62 years of age, a jeweller. Mrs N described him as rather stern, serious, and melancholy, but a man who could be very jolly with his children, to whom he is extremely attached. But she said that she had never been on intimate terms with her father:

> 'In fact, I don't really know my father, and that's partly my fault. I'm rather distant with him and I know he feels this. It's physical. [*Q*.] Yes, it's physical, I can't be on really good terms with him because I find him physically repulsive. [*Q*.] What I mean is, he has a cold look which puts me off and I just can't. And yet I know my father feels it. He calls me "sour-face". With my sister, it's different, she is much more affectionate than me. Personally, I can't, I simply *can't* give him a kiss.'

This was all said in a rather playful way.

Childhood illnesses. She had such childhood diseases as measles and chicken-pox, but could not recall any others. She remembered having had rather severe bronchitis, which was chronic up to the age of 7 years, and a tonsil-lectomy at 12 years.

Mother's gynaecological history. Her confinements were normal. Mrs N added that nothing had ever been said, but that she thought the confinements must have been normal. She knew that her mother had had her earlier children in hospital and the later ones at home. Mrs N knew that she had not been wanted, but remarked: 'My mother obviously didn't want so many children. But every time she had one, she was just as pleased. She loves children and she loves babies. Now she is very fond of her grandchildren. She's a real mother hen.'

Family background. There are two groups of brothers and sisters, the older ones, of whom one brother is 40 years of age, and the younger ones: 'My mother says, this is the second litter.' Mrs N has seven nephews and nieces. She has had a lot to do with her nephews: 'Yes, I've fed several of my nephews. I'm very fond of babies, especially little babies, and I know what it will be like when I have mine.'

The siblings to whom she feels closest are a brother of 22 and a sister of 21, with whom she grew up. She is the youngest of the family. She was questioned about this: 'Oh yes, of course it's pleasant enough. You're spoiled and made a fuss of, but you also feel that you're a burden on your parents for longer. [*Q*.] Yes, well I soon got married. But all the same, I rather resented my parents' being elderly.'

She described her adolescence: she was not terribly keen on going out, she hated gangs and had never belonged to one; similarly, she had never wanted to go to a holiday camp. She did not like crowds, and still does not like them. She was very pleased to go and live in the country, for she said

205

that she would soon grow tired of life in Paris. What she would like about Paris would be 'to come and spend money and go out a lot. Otherwise, I don't think it's very interesting, I don't like to feel in a crowd, to feel anonymous. I'm not all that keen on the place where I live; it's provincial, it's a depressing place. I much prefer the real countryside.'

She has always been with her parents except for a time when she was about 7 or 8 years old. She remembered having been left by her parents for a fortnight, on the one occasion when they went off to Haute-Savoie on holiday. She had been left with one of her sisters-in-law, and she had been quite pleased, because she was very attached to this sister-in-law, who was very fond of her. But she said that, in general, she had not liked the holidays because she had been left behind, along with her sister and her brother. She had unpleasant memories of this.

She described herself as an unruly child, but one who liked to play alone. She said that she had continued to play with dolls quite late, beyond her first period. She had some friends at school, but they were more by way of school chums. There is only one of them whom she is still seeing.

Maternal grandparents. They died shortly before her birth. She has heard little about them. She never knew her paternal grandparents.

Sex life. Mrs N had her first intercourse a few days before her marriage. Asked about this, she said:

'I hesitated. This period was rather difficult. I hesitated to give my husband a proof of love, and I didn't like going against what my mother thought. Of course, I'd never think of telling her I had sexual relations before marriage, because she would be very hurt. It's useless. Perhaps it's something she can't understand. It's better to say nothing about it. I know that I couldn't have had a prolonged affair, for then I would really have felt I was deceiving my mother and going against my whole upbringing.'

She admitted that her first intercourse had been painful: 'Well, I knew, I had been warned, and I suppose it's the same for everybody, the first time you don't enjoy it, but really, after that, I've had no further trouble.' She said that her sexual life is very satisfactory.

Feeding the baby. She knows that she was breast-fed up to 3 months. She wants to breast-feed her baby. She answered this question by saying, 'Oh yes, of course, it's more natural. I'm not going to deprive myself of that.'

Sex of the child. She will be equally pleased with a son or a daughter: 'We talk about the baby as if it were a boy, and I think if anything I'd prefer a boy, but I really don't mind at all. If it's a boy, we're going to call him Loic; that's a Breton name and my husband is a Breton. If it's a girl, we'll call her Valérie.'

206

Career ambitions. She also talked of her ambitions. She said that she would have liked to be an interior decorator, but her parents told her that this was a poorly paid occupation and that she would not be able to find work, so she had trained as a secretary.

Mrs N is a pretty, smart, well-dressed young woman. She has fair hair and green eyes. Contact is readily established with her. She verbalizes fluently, and is intelligent.

SECOND INTERVIEW WHEN 5 MONTHS PREGNANT

Same psychologist as at first interview: good contact straight away; Mrs N smiling and laughing.

Development of the pregnancy. 'My baby started moving at $3\frac{1}{2}$ months. [*Q.*] It was nice – obviously – it was quite a thrill the very first day it happened; now I like to feel him moving. [*Q.*] I have noticed that he moves a lot especially when I'm in the train coming to Paris – also when I lie down – it's always nice, never painful.'

Current symptoms. Mrs N reported rather frequent headaches. She thinks that she has a somewhat excessive craving for food during the second third of her pregnancy; some special fancies, mainly for fruit. She still has some aversions (to the smell of frying), and cannot stand the sight of a butcher's shop. As for sleeping, she enjoys restful sleep and thinks that she sleeps too much.

Dreams. She was a little reserved in revealing her dreams. She said that she frequently dreamed about her husband. Her dreams do not seem to have been unpleasant. She has had no more anxiety dreams such as occurred at the beginning of her pregnancy. At the conscious level, however, she feels more sensitive and vulnerable than at the beginning of pregnancy. She cannot bear to see detective films or scenes of violence, whereas before her pregnancy she did not consider herself at all sensitive in this respect.

Present life. She thinks about the baby a lot, but not in a concrete sense. She is preparing for the baby's arrival – the layette is ready; she has knitted it herself.

Mrs N looks forward at any moment to her husband's return. Being separated from him is causing her more and more distress. She is still living with her parents, where she is petted, spoiled, and treated like a little girl. Her mother, in particular, takes pleasure in lavishing attention on her, as if to compensate for the absence of her husband. Besides, she has always been regarded by her family as a baby.

Motherhood and Personality

Relations with parents. At this point in the interview, the parental conflict came up. She observed: 'My parents are too old, I never know whether they are right, or me.' She often feels resentful towards them. When she was little, she had been called 'the blight' or 'the pest'. 'Latterly, my mother has avoided giving me advice, because at heart she knows I don't want it. She would also like to give me hints about the baby.'

The maternal image here seems to be rather harmful objectively, because of the anxiety to which it gives rise.

When Mrs N was asked what they talked about at home, she replied, 'About business, about jewels'. She was encouraged to try to describe how she saw herself within the family. Basically, she seems to be not at all self-critical; she considers herself very good-natured. To return to her ambivalent identification with her mother, she claims that she has always liked to be smart, but 'dirty smart', as her mother called her. It was a nuisance to wash, to cut her toe nails, to wash her hair. When she was asked what else she had felt to be a nuisance, she said, 'Running errands'. It therefore appears that later, at adolescence, she had made an important narcissistic cathexis, but more in respect of dress than in respect of her body. It also seems that her only friend was simply a social acquaintance with whom she had intellectual discussions.

Emotional choice. Mrs N said that she had had a romance with her husband and that she had been secretly in love with him. At a Christmas Eve party, at which he had drunk rather a lot, he had suddenly said to her, in a loud voice, 'Will you marry me?' At the time she had refused, blushing, because she was afraid that really he was only joking. This situation lasted for a fortnight. She had been rather bewildered by it. The emotional tone of their engagement was therefore to start with that of a kind of joking episode.

When she was asked what she had known of sex, she said, laughing, 'Doesn't everyone look up the dictionary? My mother must surely have suspected it.'

Sexual relations. To start with, physical relations with her husband had been very difficult. She had a strong antipathy to kissing. And if, finally, she slept with her husband before marriage, it was 'because I didn't want the curé to go through that. I felt glad to have disobeyed them.'

She expressed the pleasure that she had taken in breaking these prohibitions and at the same time the uncomfortable feeling that she would have had if people had been able to say, on the day of her marriage, 'She'll have it tonight'. She added that she had enjoyed sex only after marriage, when she felt reassured because the mother-in-law, 'who trusted me so implicitly, was no longer in the room above', as before her marriage. She denied that she was afraid of men, but admitted that she had been very afraid of being

208

naked. She said, 'I'm very shy, it's because of my mother.' The image of the mother seems to be always oppressive. She does not seem to have any father-image. She talks of relations with him as always being rather distant. However, she seems to feel sure that he is very happy that his daughter is pregnant.

Husband. An attempt was then made to get her to say something about her husband's personality. She remarked, 'He's not like my father at all. He is emotional and demonstrative, he shows his feelings.' She spoke of his position. He is a precision engineer, a screw-cutter, and she is quite sure that he will quickly find a job.

Future. Mrs N explained that she was quite happy to stay with her parents and to look for accommodation later, but she seemed rather upset and frightened at the thought of having to adjust to housework, to looking after the baby, and to her husband. She is perhaps all the more apprehensive because hitherto her mother has looked after everything.

Preparation for childbirth. She reported that she had seen a film which had greatly impressed her, and that she was very glad to have seen it.

Attitude to her pregnancy. She feels that pregnancy is a relatively easy period, but that it restricts her activities somewhat. She has portrayed herself as a very active girl who likes to be always on the move. She had been an office girl for a woman who worked in the Marais district, and she had often had to walk long distances. She said, 'The most important thing about my pregnancy is that it has slowed me down.' She finds this slowing down pleasant.

Good contact has been maintained with this young woman. Her behaviour shows latent anxiety. Behind apparently good defences there may well be a rather childish narcissistic pattern. Her identifications seem rather confused. She denies feelings of aggression against her parents, dissociating it. The relationship with her has two sides. On the one hand, it is good-natured, warm, and a little hysteroid, and she uses charming inflexions of voice; on the other hand, one feels a certain underlying rigidity and even a rather dominating attitude.

THIRD INTERVIEW WHEN 8 MONTHS PREGNANT

A different psychologist: approach still easy; interview readily resumed by subject.

Present life and preoccupations. Mrs N's husband has just returned, his military service completed. The couple are living with her parents. They

15

have a big house, and her parents are happy with this arrangement. The couple have a room to themselves, reasonably private, and take their meals separately. They intend to remain with the parents until the child is a year old, so that they can travel. The husband has found a job, starting today. He will be earning about 800 francs per month, and, as she says, they have no rent to pay. She is no longer working. Her husband wanted to find her there when he came home, and not to find everything in confusion. Her pregnancy is 'going fine'.

'I've been wondering about circumcision if it's a boy. My parents are Jews, naturalized French subjects. My grandparents were Polish Jews. My parents are just ordinary, they aren't practising. There are extremes in the family, I keep between them. My mother-in-law is an active Catholic, very religious. My own mother is anti-religious. She believes in God but is against religious observances and against having to pay for being buried. The children were baptized, to be like everybody else. My brothers and sisters were very religious, but not me. I believe there's no smoke without fire, though – a very clever man who made people believe that he was God. I dislike ceremonies.'

The parents of Mrs N are from Warsaw. They speak Polish when they do not want their children to understand. None of the children speaks Polish. It was the grandparents who emigrated with their children to France.

Mrs N mentioned circumcision again. A sister-in-law had just had a boy. There had been much discussion about circumcision. The medical and cultural aspects had been considered, and finally it had not been done. Mrs N's husband, who is a Breton, said, 'I get on quite well without it', but he was not against it. Mrs N asked for a medical opinion on the necessity of circumcision. She was reassured on this subject. She said that she had also wondered about marital relations after the confinement:

'I've already asked a doctor who takes preparation courses. He said that 90 per cent of women were sterile until their periods started again, but I think it's better to abstain. I don't want a second baby in my arms. I want to have at least two children, and if I had plenty of money I would have another right away, but money is the essential thing and affects everything; I don't want another straight away.'

Her husband agrees with her, and in fact wants three or four children eventually.

Current symptoms. Mrs N reported obstinate constipation. She has been constipated ever since her stay in North Africa. Before that, she had normal movements.

210

Dreams. Recurrence of nightmares, which are not, she thinks, connected with her pregnancy: 'I have headaches, I sweat and wake up – but it's too complicated, I don't remember.' She was reticent at this point, and then finally reported an anxiety dream which she wanted to deny: 'I dreamed that I was losing my baby, I was having a haemorrhage. Then I woke up for good, and I felt quite relieved.'

Confinement. She is beginning to think about her confinement. Previously she had thought only about her husband's absence: 'I think I'll manage, without getting worked up and without getting afraid. It isn't nice to be afraid.' Several of her sisters-in-law had prepared confinements which went well. But, as she says, she has a vivid imagination: 'When I got letters from my husband, they took four days to arrive, and I used to wonder if he was still alive when I got them.'

When she was at school, it was the same. She was frightened when she had an examination – she had a frightful attack of nerves. Once she was inside she was all right. She knew it was silly, because she was a good pupil, but it was due to pride: 'My sister did well. I wanted to be like her.' She added with a smile, 'It's a good stimulus.'

The baby. She has been thinking of possible defects: 'I would be surprised if there were any, since there have never been any in the family. I mean, born deaf or blind. Once, in particular, I wondered, because I had been to see my sister-in-law, and one of her children had measles or something like that, but I wasn't afraid for long.'

Health. At this point, she spoke about skin trouble. She has acne:

'I have a very fatty skin. It began when I was about 14 or 15. But I deal with it more effectively now. I dry my skin. One of my two brothers suffers a lot from acne. He is 40, and he has it still. He ate the wrong things when he was young. He suffered from hunger right through the war. My sister also suffers a bit from acne. We all tend to have weak lungs, we get that from my mother. It's irritation rather than a real lung disease. My lungs are weaker. I had bronchitis when I was quite young. They gave me a spray. My mother took good care of me, and it never got very serious. I am getting terribly fat at the moment.'

And she asked if she would get slim again after she had her baby: 'These are selfish details,' she said, 'but after all . . .' She is on a salt-free diet at present: 'I believe it's better for the confinement. I live fifteen miles from Paris . . . I have a half-hour journey. I would like to leave home in good time, neither too early nor too late. What should I do? My husband is working during visiting hours. Will he be able to come to see me all the same?'

Sex life. 'We both feel frustrated.' She blushed. They had not resumed sexual relations since the seventh month, when the husband came home. This is being careful, 'so as not to tire me or the baby'. She had not asked for advice, but had consulted books: 'In LP's book, you are advised to be careful. Dr L's book is much better, but it doesn't mention this point, so I think perhaps it can't be of much importance. Anyway, as far as we're concerned, it's to avoid getting tired.' She said that she felt very frustrated by this interruption of sexual life: 'We were used to living together. We're just like animals as far as that goes. We need it, it's natural just as for animals.' She reported a full sex life, with orgasm. 'I took a long time to get used to it. My mother was prudish. She must have been like me before, considering her physical type. All that sort of thing was regarded as not fit to mention. It was mostly shyness. It wasn't easy to get used to it.'

Early development. On the question of learning to walk: 'I don't know, my mother told me but I can't remember. I wasn't late, I was never late in any way.'

Cleanliness. 'Until I was 14, my mother played war with me. I was dirty and untidy. I finally gave in.' She was asked to say just in what way she was dirty: 'Well, we lived in the country and they didn't bother much with me. Until I was 2, I dirtied my nappies. I had mumps, tonsillitis, 'flu, the usual illnesses. I never had whooping-cough. But I always coughed a lot, which comes to the same thing.'

Background. She grew up during the war. Because of its Jewish origin, Mrs N's family went into hiding. She reported that her third brother was at present suffering from a nervous breakdown. She said: 'It's a result of the war. He is married, and he's having trouble with his wife. He feels overwhelmed, a failure. It's the war that wore him out. He had responsibilities too young. He was 21 at the beginning of the war. The family was more or less scattered. It's afterwards that you feel it.'

Then Mrs N spoke of difficulties at school during her childhood. She had had no girl friends except one, who was a very intelligent girl; she herself liked boys better: 'Women are always making a fuss. I don't feel jealous when I see a beautiful woman.'

The impression of intelligence and charm was maintained. The anxiety noticed during the first two interviews appeared more clearly during the third interview. The change of psychologist certainly had something to do with it, but, more important, towards the end of the pregnancy, both ego strength and the strength of defences seem to have lost in effectiveness, and released a degree of deep-lying anxiety connected with cultural traditions and parental identifications.

212

MRS N'S CONFINEMENT

The observer was called at 1.15 a.m. to a patient four fingers dilated. He arrived at 1.30. The patient was then fully dilated. She had gone into hospital at midnight.

Observation therefore started later than for other cases, because of a rapid labour and a telephone call which had been unavoidably delayed.

The labour ward was quiet. The observer found the patient lying on her back, apparently, at first glance, having established a very good relationship with the midwife. She was calm although rather anxious, and salivating freely. She seemed to be quite well controlled, yet near the limit of her control.

Her eyes were half-closed. She seemed to be looking out through the slits. At this point, she was placed in the dorsal position with her feet in stirrups, and said, 'This is it, I've to bear down?' in a questioning tone. That was the first bearing-down effort. She creased her face in a rather comic grin, and expelled air with a noise like an aeroplane. She seemed preoccupied, bore down not quite low enough, but then proceeded quite well. After bearing down, she answered questions without moving her head, but with a kind of peevish eagerness and objectivity. She said that it was better now that she was bearing down, and that she was hardly suffering any more. The second time, she apparently bore down very effectively. She then said that she had had pains especially in the lower abdomen, but also in the back, and that she had had pains in the back continuously for more than a week. The third time, she continued to bear down very effectively, with a comic pout which made her lips look thicker. She was, however, slightly cyanosed. She continued to answer without looking at the observer and showed no special reaction to the questions, but she showed a kind of over-concern, each time repeating 'What do you mean?' Finally, she said that she felt the baby descending. It was still rather painful. The midwife informed her at that point that it was the stage of issue. She answered, 'Ye-ess', drawing out the 'e', and took off the mask with anxious and abrupt haste. The baby was born at 1.50. Expulsion had therefore required only seven or eight bearing-down efforts and had lasted fifteen minutes.

There was no disorganization of behaviour at the stage of issue, but only a narrowing of the field of consciousness with an underlying anxiety which one could feel coming to the surface.

She obeyed very well the midwife's instruction to stop bearing down, thought for a moment of a possible episiotomy, and gave a frantic panting breath, groaning a little. She watched her baby emerge, first through half-closed eyes, then with a wondering smile. When she was told that it was a boy, she said 'Frederick'. She sat up to look at him and asked with a fairly clear voice that his face should be turned towards her. Her gestures showed

213

great maternal tenderness. She sat up of her own accord and said, 'Oh! Oh! Oh! He makes a nice noise, he's funny. I'm not surprised, because I've seen them in films.'

She had to check the identification bracelet,[1] and showed no special reaction. She seemed both a little bewildered and a little lost. 'Have I to bear down?', she asked of the placental delivery. The latter occurred ten minutes later without any contractions and very easily.

Her account of the confinement was as follows:

'Dilatation is much more unpleasant than delivery, it hurts, it hurts frightfully, whereas the actual delivery isn't too bad. It was uncomfortable having to hold myself in. It was a relief to bear down. I didn't feel his actual arrival and I certainly thought it would be much worse. At the beginning, the pain is a nuisance, it's severe, it gets you down and takes all your strength away, you just can't get about any more.'

When the baby was brought back again, she laughed a little and said, 'He's not pretty but he's sweet; his tummy looks odd. I can't imagine that I've got a baby, I just can't believe it.' At this point she had a mild general reaction with trembling. She spoke willingly, in a careful and pleasant voice: 'For nine months I've been thinking about it. It got unreal, and now there it is.' She had expected her confinement only on the following morning. She had not felt any apprehension: 'We had been so well prepared, and had so much crammed into our heads.' All the same, she had not expected to have no pain at all: 'Breathing helped a lot, and prevented me from bearing down; it kept me busy and prevented me from twisting about in all directions. It didn't have any direct effect on the pain.' And when she had the fit of trembling by way of reaction, she said, 'I've got the shakes, it gets on my nerves.' She agreed that the staff had been important, but that was all.

She had two small stitches for a slight perineal tear, and reacted mildly to this. She complained of the tremors in her legs, saying, 'How silly these legs are', using a childish expression. She took refuge in panting, and said, 'That helps'. She showed a somewhat ingenuous humour: '*C'est une maison de haute couture ici.*'[2] When she was told to relax, she threw her arms behind her. 'Not too much', the midwife said, 'it makes you bleed.' 'Oh, all right', said the patient – 'I'm thirsty.' She was given a little drink. Her relations with the staff were tinged with humour. When she was being washed, she was told: 'It's soothing, it does you good,' whereupon she laughed gently.

[1] Every baby is given a bracelet with his or her name on it before the cord is cut.

[2] *Translator's note:* The play on words is impossible to translate. The phrase, of course, means: 'This is a high-class dressmaking establishment'; but also, if taken literally, it could be rendered: 'a high-class sewing establishment'.

214

'When I think that my sister was fifteen hours in labour! I had my first regular contractions, close together, about 7.30 p.m. and that was very painful. I did my breathing exercises right away. I didn't think that it was time, they were too close. I went on with my dinner, and then I went to bed. I couldn't settle down. I had the shakes. I got a hot water bottle, and the warmth did me good. My husband and my parents were there. I was glad that my husband was there. The others didn't matter . . .'

This was said in a tone of hostility: 'My mother no longer gives me advice because she knows that I don't take it. My elder sister had a figure like a little girl. I don't know what that means, but I think that's why she had a bad confinement. My sister went to live in America two years ago.'

To recapitulate, in this case, dilatation was fairly brief, taking about five hours, with almost continuous pains in the lower abdomen. 'I told my husband to telephone for the ambulance and in the middle of the journey the waters broke. I didn't want to arrive late.' She arrived at the hospital at ten minutes after midnight: 'I had difficulty in walking, but it was all right, I felt more confident.'

She was examined by a midwife who put her into the labour ward. She was then two fingers dilated. She reported that she at once felt at ease, and asked for something to be put under her knees. As she continued to tremble, she took deep breaths to try to stop it. She said now that she felt very proud, and that it upset her to feel herself trembling: 'The desire to bear down was nothing,' she said, 'but what was hard was that I was not to bear down. It was like wanting to go to the toilet, but not in the same place.' She gave an embarrassed and rather precious and affected little giggle – 'like too strong a laxative which makes you feel you're going to be turned inside out like a glove', she said.

The impression given was of a fundamentally sound young woman, a little artificial, prim and self-assertive, but able to make herself agreeable, a little affected but well adjusted, who established an excellent immediate maternal relationship with her baby.

'I never let up. I did my exercises like anything since June,' she said; and technically, she had mastered the breathing techniques extremely well. 'As far as relaxation was concerned,' she said, 'I was relaxed all right, but not completely because I am very nervous. I get tensed up and I remain very self-conscious.' Analgesia was therefore only partial, with pains which were distressing particularly because of their recurrence. These pains seemed to the patient to have a certain significance and a kind of necessity. 'The staff were very good to me,' she said. She seemed very positive and direct, but also very tense.

She asked if she could add another name, and she chose Loic, which is Breton for Louis, because her husband is a Breton – but not for a first name

215

because it would be odd. 'Frederick? I like that, it sounds Scandinavian, I like it.' At this point, she behaved like a younger daughter of a good family:

'I heard the midwife when she said that it was coming, and I could hardly believe it, because I thought it would be worse. At the stage of issue, I felt nothing. Inside, it was a very intense feeling, much greater than anything I've ever felt. In fact, it was tremendous. I feel rather grown-up. I was always regarded as the baby because I was the eighth.'

She therefore had a very enriching experience. 'When I have a baby, I shall have proved myself', she thought. Her baby had not yet been brought back, but she said, 'That doesn't matter'.

To conclude, Mrs N showed a defence involving laughing and grinning; she was tense, with a childish voice, and a little tyrannical. 'He was moving up to the last moment; I was very much on edge today. I was covering the cradle with cloth and I burned some things in the kitchen. Usually, I am quite calm,' she said.

The impression she is likely to retain of her confinement is one of short duration, of inevitable pain, which, nevertheless, was less than she had expected, of an efficient staff, and of a maturing experience.

SUMMARY

To summarize, Mrs N was the eighth child of a family, who was not at first wanted, and was then brought up by a rather rigid mother in an atmosphere of duty, and above all in a social climate of insecurity (ethnic problems). She had difficulty in establishing good parental identifications.

Basically, however, she was fairly secure. She overemphasized her maturity in order to be of equal status with the others. She is a narcissistic woman whose sound defences enabled her to overcome the anxiety associated with childbirth, to assimilate preparation well, and therefore to have a successful confinement.

Despite her narcissism, she had a good maternal attitude and at once established a good relation to her baby.

If one wished to classify Mrs N in psychiatric terms, one might say that she had a hysterical-phobic personality.

Her total negativity score was 21, which put her in the middle group of the women prepared for childbirth. According to this average level of negativity, she should have had an average confinement, i.e. one in class two. In fact, her confinement was sufficiently successful (score of 15) to be included in class one.

This is a case of a woman whose negativity was 'neutralized' by preparation because a good system of defences was reinforced, and also because

216

she reacted to preparation with the desire to make progress with it and succeed, just as, at a younger age, she had wanted to be a good pupil.

CONFINEMENT RECORD

00.10   Full-term pregnancy
         Foetal heart heard; fully engaged head
         Cervix dilated two fingers
         Enema
00.50   1 mg. of 20 per cent methionate intravenously
01.30   Dilatation almost complete; foetal heart heard
01.40   Dilatation complete
         Expulsive efforts
01.50   Normal childbirth at term
         Left occipito-anterior engagement of the head
         Release of the head in the occipito-posterior position
         Birth of a boy, immediate crying
          Weight, 7 lb. 5 oz.; length, 19 inches
02.00   Normal and apparently complete delivery of the placenta, weighing
         19 oz.
         Two stitches

PREPARATION RECORD

First phase: taking up of cervix and dilatation to three fingers

   Very frequent uterine contractions; very rapid dilatation
   Patient well controlled
   Methionate

Second phase: from three fingers to full dilatation

   (a) *Psychological reaction* – patient calm
   (b) *Muscular relaxation* – quite good
   (c) *Breathing* – very good
   (d) Shows signs of suffering, but well controlled

Third phase: expulsion

   (a) *Psychological reaction* – patient disciplined and active
   (b) *Expulsive efforts* – very good
   (c) *Delivery of the head* – rather difficult

Subjective assessment by patient

   She found dilatation painful (earlier lumbar pain)

217

Comments

Labour – 5 hours; expulsion – 15 minutes
Behaviour on the whole very good
Rapid labour, painful dilatation
Patient calm, pleasant, and most anxious to cooperate
Expulsion very good

G. GAYLE STEPHENS, M.D.
3232 East Pine
Wichita, Kansas   67208

CONFINEMENT GRID

Stage	Obstetrical index	Pain	Behaviour	Pain + Behaviour
Dilatation	1	3	1	4
Transition	1	4	2	6
Part total	2	7	3	10
Expulsion	1	2	1	3
Issue	2	1	1	2
Part total	3	3	2	5
Total over 4 stages	5	10	5	15

Activity: +1

Relations with staff: Quality 2
                       Intensity 2

Relation to baby: Quality 1
                   Intensity 1

Preparation techniques:

	Use	Effectiveness
Breathing	1	2
Relaxation	2	2
Bearing down	1	1

Explanatory comments:
Confinement successful from point of view of behavioural control, and therefore from point of view of preparation.

Successful issue, perfect from the point of view of preparation, although obstetrically a little difficult.

NEGATIVITY GRID

Name: *Mrs N*   Case Number: *X*

I. HISTORY	Childhood				Puberty-Adolescence				Adulthood			
	Mother	*Father*	*Husband*	*Others*	*Mother*	*Father*	*Husband*	*Others*	*Mother*	*Father*	*Husband*	*Others*
A Individual pathology												
(a) traumas												
(b) symptoms			+				+					
B Womanhood												
(a) gynaecological pathology												
(b) inadequate information												
(c) negative incidents							+					
(d) difficulties concerning womanhood											+	
C Family background												
(a) traumas	+											
(b) pathology		+										+
(c) interpersonal difficulties	+					+				+		
(d) disturbances in family environment								+				
D Social life												
(a) economic difficulties												
(b) difficulties over social adjust-							+				+	

II. PREGNANCY

	Stage I	Stage II	Hospital adjustment
A General pathology			Remarks
B Gynaecological-obstetrical pathology			
C Psychosomatic symptoms		+	
D Difficulties concerning womanhood and motherhood			
E Psychopathological symptoms			I = 12
(a) concerning woman		+	II = 9
(b) concerning baby			Total = 21
(c) specific symptoms		++	
F Character and behaviour disorders			

	Stage I		Stage II	
	Mother	Family	Mother	Family
G Family troubles	Husband	Husband's family	Husband	Husband's family
	+		+	+
			+ (Mother)	+ (Family)

| H Social and economic difficulties | + | | |

NOTES ON MRS N'S NEGATIVITY GRID

I. *Negativity in personal history*

A(a) col. 1 tonsillectomy
 (b) col. 2 illness (bronchitis)
B(b) col. 2 not informed by mother
 (d) col. 3 guilt feelings towards mother
C(b) col. 3 brother's neurasthenia
 (c) col. 1 mother and father during childhood
 (c) col. 2 father and social relationships ⎫ interpersonal
              during adolescence   ⎬ difficulties
 (c) col. 3 father during adulthood ⎭
D(b) cols. 2 difficulties of social adjustment during
        & 3 adolescence and adulthood

II. *Negativity during pregnancy*

C   col. 2 headaches – pains
E(b) col. 2 fantasies of abnormality
 (c) col. 2 anxiety dreams
G   cols. 1 difficulties with husband's family over religion
       & 2 and possible circumcision
              difficulties with husband over separation
              conflict with own parents
H   col. 1 lack of accommodation

Second Case-history

This is a case of a young woman whose previous history and personality are of a very different kind. Here we have a woman who refused preparation for various reasons, some contingent (work and holidays), others more deep-lying, as will be shown in the third interview and the summary.

MRS K

FIRST INTERVIEW WHEN 3 MONTHS PREGNANT

Civil status and socio-economic status. Mrs K lives near the hospital. She is a manicurist, 28 years of age, and has been married for three years. She is a big dark woman, well groomed and elegantly dressed, heavily made up and attractive. When she was asked the date of her marriage, she took out her marriage certificate, saying with an interesting air of justifying herself, 'This is so you can see that it's true . . . '

Her husband is 31 years of age and is a commercial representative. The couple's financial resources are difficult to estimate, since their incomes are somewhat variable (the husband earns between 500 and 600 francs, and the woman herself earns between 300 and 400 francs per month).

Accommodation. The young couple are currently living with Mr K's father. They have done so since their marriage and see no reason to change: 'He has a big flat – it was he who proposed the arrangement. He is 62 – a very nice man . . . It's just like having our own place. We take our meals with him . . . But now, its more as though he were living with us.'

From the beginning of the interview, in which good contact was established, Mrs K concerned herself with the problem of her pregnancy.

Menstrual cycle and sex life. When she first missed a period, it did not occur to Mrs K that she might be pregnant: 'At the beginning, until I was nearly 20, I had very regular periods, but after that age they became irregular and very painful.' On the first day of her periods, she vomited, fainted, and sometimes suffered from dizziness: 'Everything went round and I couldn't stand upright . . . It was terrible . . . I had pains all over.'

Talking about this dysmenorrhoea, Mrs K said in a very aggressive tone that she had had hormone treatment for it, and blamed this for the fact that she had developed hypertrichosis, to which, psychologically, she reacted badly.

Mrs K had had her first period at the age of 14, and menstruation had been free from pain and normal in amount. She spontaneously associated the appearance of menstruation with the beginning of her sex life. As soon

222

as she reached the question of her sex life, she changed her attitude and assumed the tone of someone trying to justify herself:

'Yes, I had sexual relations, but of course, at that time I felt sure that I would get engaged. I knew what I was doing, and so I was able to let myself go. I don't hold with that, you know. I would never have slept with a man without being engaged, but it happened because at the time I was engaged; otherwise, you know, he had been wanting to sleep with me for a long time, but I didn't want to.'

Mrs K was married at the age of 25½. She would seem to have had amenorrhoea for thirty-one months before her marriage. [Q.] 'No, I never thought of it for a moment. I was quite sure that I wasn't pregnant. A woman who doesn't want a baby doesn't get pregnant.'

At this point, she was asked what method of contraception they used. She stammered and explained, blushing, that her husband withdrew and then she washed herself out. She described this process with some pleasure and without embarrassment and explained that she washed herself thoroughly and as far in as she could, so that she was sure that it was effective. She said again:

'I was absolutely certain that I wasn't pregnant, but I did go to see a gynaecologist, and he said, "You're pregnant" when I told him I hadn't had a period for three months. Finally, he agreed that I wasn't mad, that I knew what I was talking about, and that I wasn't pregnant. I felt well, *I wasn't having any trouble*. Besides, if I had been pregnant, I would have been ill, whereas in fact there was nothing wrong with me. [Q.] Yes, I think that when you are pregnant, you are ill. It's not inevitably so, I don't feel particularly ill, but all the same, I would have known if I had been pregnant, and in fact I wasn't. I wasn't tired, I felt perfectly all right, only I wasn't having my periods.'

She had a hormone-induced menstrual cycle and her periods returned. This spell of amenorrhoea occurred a year and a half before her marriage.

Attitude to pregnancy now. At the present time, she definitely welcomed her pregnancy, and commented:

'I myself wanted a child, in fact, I have wanted one for a long time; it was my husband who didn't want it. I really did want a baby this time. The gynaecologist explained to me the times at which conception was most likely, and I took my temperature, but my husband got fed up with all the bother with taking temperatures, and, indeed, I did all I could to become pregnant. And every month, my period was there again. I was in despair. My husband, on the other hand, was very pleased. I was making him give me this baby, and my husband did what I wanted to please me, but he always gave the impression that he didn't expect anything to happen and didn't think I would become pregnant . . . Then in December, I had a very small menstrual loss, and I thought I might possibly be pregnant, because my mother, when she had me, started her pregnancy by having periods for two months. I said to myself, "That's it, I'm like my mother, I'm pregnant!" That was in December. In January, I missed my period.'

Symptoms. Mrs K said that during January she was very tired, sleeping very deeply and long, and she said that she had pain in her breasts. This pain was described in rather extreme terms:

'I couldn't bear to have anyone touch me. Even if someone just brushed against me, I yelled, it was so sore. That went on for two months. But I wasn't worried, I had been warned. My sister had the same thing when she was pregnant. She told me, "It starts in the breasts, you'll see, you'll have a lot of pain in the breasts." '

During January (the first month of her pregnancy), Mrs K vomited a few times. She said that during the next month she felt very tired, and suffered from hypersomnia and constipation.

Mrs K is now in the third month of her pregnancy. She said that she was still tired, and used the expression, 'dragging myself along'. She said that she didn't feel at all like working, that she was very nervous and irritable, and that she was very apt to argue with her husband, which must be unpleasant for him, but she was hypersensitive and her nerves were on edge.

She reported that she sometimes vomited when she was tired, but that on the whole this did not happen very often. Other symptoms included occasional headaches and hypersomnia as from the beginning of the pregnancy; her constipation was cured. She also reported rather copious leucorrhoea, which she had never had before.

Dreams. 'Yes, I dreamed quite recently, a week ago, that I had a lovely little girl, and that she was really mine. I dreamed that because I had read stories about the substitution of babies in the papers and had been quite affected by them.'

Husband's attitude. Mrs K had waited until the end of the second month before seeking medical care for her pregnancy:

'Yes, I preferred to wait two months to be sure. My gynaecologist is a woman, I would rather be examined by a woman, I find it less embarrassing. When I got back home my husband was watching for me out of the window, and at once I made a sign to say I was pregnant, and I saw that he was horrified. He said, "I hope you'll get an abortion." As far as I was concerned, there was no question of that. I don't think he really meant it, but he may have said it just to see how I would react. I was really very pleased. My husband wasn't yet reconciled to my pregnancy, because he is apt to be jealous and rather possessive, and he may think that when I have a baby I won't pay much attention to him any more. But I've tried to explain to him that it's not the same thing and that I need a child. Anyway, I know he's not very pleased about my being pregnant. He was dismayed at first, but he's beginning to get used to it. If I hadn't wanted the child and had wanted to have an abortion, he would have been very pleased. It's true, of course, that he did everything to make me pregnant, but he didn't think it would actually happen. Yes, he thought I would be sterile, and that I would be pleased if I were, because he didn't want to feel opposed to me. In the end, he was quite nice about it. He does more or less what I want.'

Choice of hospital. Mrs K came to this hospital simply because it is the nearest one to where she lives and is included on the list of hospitals recommended by the Social Insurance. She said that, of course, if she had had the money, she would have got her own medical attendant to supervise her pregnancy.

Preparation for childbirth. She did not seem to know quite what the method involves. She said that one of her customers had spoken to her about it and had been very satisfied with it, and that she was going to find out about it first; if it really looked as if it helped one to suffer less, she would be delighted.

Fantasy life. She said that she was very worried and afraid of things going wrong, afraid of dying; in this connexion she reported that, when she was having her painful periods, she had been told that she had an ovarian cyst and now she was concerned about it. At this point, she described again her contraceptive precautions and said that in the course of these, she 'had touched a kind of swelling, a long way inside the vagina'. She described herself as 'a worrier' and said that if anything was wrong she always thought the worst, both for others and for herself. In this connexion, she said that she had a friend who had a little pimple which was getting bigger; she had thought that her friend might have cancer (though she had not said so to her). She observed that she reacted more or less like that all the time: when anything was wrong, she feared the worst, and with regard to her own confinement, she was afraid of dying.

Early development. She does not know much about her early life, and said that people had never talked to her about it. She does, however, know that she was breast-fed for a very long time: 'Yes I remember, when my elder sister must have been 5, I was still on the breast.'

225

16

Motherhood and Personality

Breast-feeding. Mrs K does not want to breast-feed her baby, for narcissistic reasons. She remarked ,'It spoils one's breasts, that's partly why I don't want to do it.' She looked embarrassed and blushed. She explained that she wanted to bring up the child herself and that she was going to stop working; this was something else which she had had to get her husband to agree to, because he wanted her to go on working. She said: 'As soon as I was pregnant, I raised the question. I told him that if I had a baby, I wasn't going to hand it over to anybody else; I want it completely to myself, and I won't work any more. For all I earn, it's not worth while paying a nurse.'

She went on to explain that her husband had now accepted her decision, but that he wasn't at all pleased about it.

Childhood illnesses. She said she had had tonsillitis. In fact, this occurred only twice, but it seems to have had a psychological effect on her. She regarded it as the most serious illness she had had. Having previously said 'No, I wasn't ill', she went on, 'I never had anything much, just minor illnesses. Oh, I remember, I had bad tonsillitis.' She also revealed that she had had measles, mumps, erysipelas at the age of $10\frac{1}{2}$, and pleurisy when she was 21, which was connected with emotional difficulties with her fiancé.

Mother. Her mother is 58. She belongs to a farming family. Mrs K sees her once a year, for she had left her home district quite early to come to work in Paris. She thinks that her mother must now have passed the menopause, but she said that her mother had suffered from it for a long time just when she herself was getting married. Her mother wrote to her frequently at this time explaining that she felt tired, that she had serious haemorrhages and that she was obliged to stay in bed. Mrs K said that her mother had certainly had easy pregnancies and normal confinements, which took place in the country, at home. She remarked: 'There was a doctor who should have come, but I know, because I've been told so, that my mother's confinements were very short. It was my grandmother who delivered us. She was the midwife.'

Family background. She indicated that she had a step-brother of 37 years of age, her father's son by a previous marriage. Her father was a widower when he married her mother, her mother having been divorced. They both had a child of approximately the same age, and Mrs K therefore had both a step-brother and a step-sister of 37, but she referred to them as a step-brother and a sister. When she was asked to repeat this, she said, 'Yes, she is my sister, she's my mother's daughter.'

The rest of the family consists of Mrs K herself and a real sister of 21, who lives in the country, and is married with two children. She said that this second sister had a boy 5 years old and another younger boy (one year old), and had just had a miscarriage at three months.

226

Here she explained the family difficulties there had been because her sister (step-sister) got pregnant. According to her sister's own account, she was raped one day when she was returning home on her bicycle, but the incident was confused, and Mrs K does not seem to be very clear about it. She knows that her parents were very shaken, and that it was never discovered who the father of the child really was.

Mrs K left home when she was about 15½ years old. She said, 'I was never meant to live in the country or to be a farmer. My mother understood that perfectly.' She then described her mother as a very understanding and intelligent woman who had a very close and confidential relationship with her daughter.

Emotional and sexual life. When she was very young, Mrs K had been engaged for the first time to a boy from her own village, but after a time she had refused to marry him. Her first affair after that was with an officer in the regular army who promised to marry her but who, as she found out later, had no intention of doing so, as he was already living with another woman.

Her third affair was with her future husband. She very readily told the story of this affair. She met him at a fair and he invited her to go on a merry-go-round with him, and then she saw him again. At first it was just a flirtation and she enjoyed it. Then he wanted to sleep with her; she refused and began to talk of marriage. He took a long time to make up his mind. As soon as they were engaged (she was 20), they had sexual relations, and he refused marriage on the ground that his father did not approve because she came from a social class inferior to his. This went on for five years. She said that she had suddenly had enough of it. A year before her marriage, she had been in a state of great anxiety over her position, and at this point she got pleurisy and went home. He followed her, and they got engaged and settled the date of the wedding.

This account was all very confused. Mrs K obscured important facts among very minor details and it was impossible to note everything. Her whole emotional life indicates a certain childishness, the incidents being recounted like confidences, supported by the advice received from her palmist, etc.

Sex life. She spoke of her first sexual relations as mildly painful. She was a little disillusioned by sex. She was not innocent, and she knew what happened, but, even so, she had had a different notion of love. It did emerge, however, that she had soon come to enjoy intercourse, though it was not clear whether her pleasure was derived from the vagina or from the clitoris. She added, 'Yes, it's very important for me, and this is proved by the fact that when I don't have it I get ill.' She said that when she did not have sexual relations, she felt sick and had headaches: 'I really do need it.' She was certainly blooming. The couple appear to have intercourse very frequently.

Sex of the baby. She does not mind in the least whether it is a boy or a girl.

To summarize, good rapport was established with a narcissistic, rather immature woman who likes to talk about herself in a superficial way.

SECOND INTERVIEW WHEN 5½ MONTHS PREGNANT

Same psychologist: good rapport was established straight away.

Mrs K explained that she was unable to come to her previous appointment because she is free only on Mondays. She is a manicurist and makes use of her day off.

Current symptoms. When it was remarked that her skin looked rather blotchy, she said that when she had her periods she always got blotches like that, and that it was worse just then. She reported that she had had several slight nose-bleeds, especially when she blew her nose, and that her gums had been bleeding since she had become pregnant. When she talked about her work, she said that she tended to feel some nausea when there was a smell of permanent waving or tinting, but she could still do her job quite easily because she was seated and it did not tire her too much.

Vomiting had stopped at the beginning of the fourth month. She has a good appetite, whereas at the beginning of her pregnancy she had a poorer appetite; but if she eats too much, she has pains in her stomach. She has not got too fat.

She had been constipated from the beginning of her pregnancy, but is no longer so. She explained that she took a laxative, and asked whether that might do the baby any harm. An attempt was made to see whether she had any other worries about the baby. She acknowledged that she was worried about the times when she dined with her father-in-law. Her father-in-law provided good wine at dinner, and she enjoyed it, but wondered whether it might not be bad for the baby.

Future at work. Mrs K was going to leave her hairdressing salon at the end of July and would prefer not to return to work. Her husband would prefer her to go on working, but she herself would rather look after her baby.

In general, she had been sleeping well, but sometimes her sleep was interrupted by painful cramps in the legs. She complained of backache when she sat all day doubled up on her stool at the shop.

Dreams. She was very reluctant to relate her dreams. Then she said, with obvious anxiety, 'I dreamed that my husband was deceiving me with another woman. I had this dream on Saturday night.' This nightmare seems to have given rise to considerable anxiety.

Relationship with husband. She revealed that her husband, of his own accord, had stopped having sexual relations since the third month of her pregnancy.

228

He was afraid of doing her harm and also, when she reassured him about this, he explained that he did not have any great desire. She commented, 'Yes, I'm very vexed about that, and rather fed up.' She said that she herself felt extremely unsatisfied:

'I tried to make him understand that it doesn't do any harm, that it can't hurt me and that it wouldn't tire me, but then I realized that he just didn't like the thought of it. I can't really understand it, because at three months I wasn't very big, I didn't have a big belly. I couldn't understand it and I began to worry. I even told him so. I was afraid that he was going with other women, but he said he wasn't, and I think I can trust him. However, I don't see why he feels intercourse to be intolerable. But then, you know, my husband is just a child, you can't explain anything to him. He's 32, but he behaves like a boy of 14 or 15.'

She described him as a lively, noisy fellow, and what she called 'heedless'. She said that he was incapable of accepting responsibility, and that he would always remain a child; that he paid her a fair amount of attention, asking her how she was, but showing no interest whatever in the baby. He did not want to hear it mentioned. She remarked, 'Often he says to me, "It just can't be, it isn't my doing." '

He has therefore rejected the pregnancy completely and does not want to hear a word about it. Mrs K explained that when she was getting the layette ready and embroidering sheets, she showed them to him and he said, 'What do you want to show me all that for? He won't need all that, why do it? There's plenty of time to think about it,' etc.

She stated that her husband had not had any affairs before marriage, and that she herself was very highly sexed. She was clearly frustrated by his continued denial to her of sexual satisfaction. She observed, 'No, he wasn't disappointed with me sexually. On the contrary, he sometimes used to say, "Relax, for goodness' sake, or you'll do for me." '

On the question of whether her husband was having any extramarital affairs, she said that she was almost sure that he wasn't. In a very involved account, she explained that her husband had nocturnal emissions but that she missed her sex life terribly and suffered greatly from abstinence: 'Sometimes I try to insist, but really there isn't anything I can do, he simply doesn't care about it any more; and yet I'm not ugly.'

With regard to her confinement, she said that she definitely would not want her husband to be present, and that in any case he would not want to be there. 'My husband already finds me repulsive since I became pregnant, so what would he be like if he saw me having my baby?'

In connexion with her pregnancy, she remarked that they never mentioned the child between themselves and it was almost a forbidden topic. When she told her husband that the baby had moved, he said, 'You've dreamed it, it's impossible, it's impossible.' He reacted with disgust. Apparently he had tried to feel the baby moving with his hand, and had recoiled in revulsion. Her husband's attitude very much disturbed Mrs K. For her, the most serious problem appeared to be the denial of sexual satisfaction since the beginning of her pregnancy.

There was a long discussion about her husband. She described him as a lazy child whom she more or less had to force to work. They are living with her father-in-law, to whom she is very attached. The son (her husband) is still very dependent on his father, whom he asks for money. The father-in-law is delighted with this situation and the couple have no independent social life. The father-in-law takes them out, to the cinema, to dinner,etc. An attempt was made to show Mrs K that the childishness for which she criticized her husband was aggravated by his dependent role in relation to his father. She had indeed been aware of this and had tried to get accommodation of their own. When they were ready to buy this flat, however, her husband had not the courage to tell his father. One day she informed her father-in-law by telephone at his office. It was a great shock for him. He did finally accept it, but then told his son, 'If you take a flat of your own and leave me alone, I'll marry again.' The son was very much against his father's remarrying: 'My husband told me, "I won't have another woman in what was my mother's house. I simply won't have my father remarrying. If it's the flat against my father's marriage, that's that! We'll stay where we are and live with father."'

That, in fact, is the crux of the problem. Mr K had lost his mother when he was 21 years of age. He has a serious mother-fixation. His wife is well aware of this, and avoids the mother problem. She justified herself as follows:

'When I mentioned his mother and tried to find out what she had died of, he immediately began to cry. He said his mother had been the most wonderful woman in the world and he refused to speak about her, it hurt him so much. It's something the same for my father-in-law, too. Personally, it seems to me perfectly normal for him to marry again, but his son is dead against it. Now things have settled down again and we'll never have our flat, we'll go on living with my father-in-law until he dies; seeing that if we leave he will get married again.'

Father-in-law. He is 62 and in good health. He has a good position in the civil service, and has spoiled his son. The two men had been shattered by the death of their wife and mother. Mrs K said that her husband had never been away from his father; he had always remained with his parents. An attempt was made to get a clearer understanding of this triangle of the woman between these two men. Mrs K said that she was very fond of her father-in-law and that he was a perfect gentleman and very kind. Sometimes there were arguments between father and son, and when this happened she did not interfere but left them to work it out themselves:

'When that happens, I simply have to go away; they are both stubborn, I never know who gives in, but anyway, it's easy for my husband. He knows that his father's greatest pleasure is to give him money. He spoils us both dreadfully, but I realize that kind of thing isn't good for my husband; and when we have the baby I want to give up my work, which I can quite readily do, and I'll explain to my husband that he must work harder, since he has a wife and child to keep.'

Social life. The couple have in fact no social life. Mrs K had two women friends in whom she was greatly disappointed. She explained that they were jealous of her and that one of them had tried to seduce her husband. She was in the process of getting a divorce and made eyes at Mrs K's husband. This woman had become a nude dancer in a night club, and Mrs K regarded her as a 'fallen woman' and would not go out with her any more. Mrs K has cut herself off from her friends, her husband has none either, and the couple are therefore restricted to their relations with the father-in-law.

Sex of the baby. She would like a boy with blue eyes like her husband, and her husband would rather have a daughter. Mrs K would like to call a daughter Nadine because she likes the name, but her husband insists that she be called Éliane, which was his mother's name; so it is decided that if the baby is a girl, she will be called Éliane. A Christian name for a boy has not yet been decided.

Movements of baby. Mrs K felt the baby moving at the end of the fourth month. She said that she was lying down and felt very tired at the time. It was in the evening, and she was very thrilled. She told her husband, who said that it wasn't possible and reacted with revulsion, as has already been stated. Mrs K remarked, 'It was funny to start with, but now that I am getting used to it, it's nicer.'

Upbringing. At this point, the interview returned to Mrs K's past history:

'I had an idea that a rather strict upbringing would be a good thing, but mummy said, "Wait and see", and it's true, I've changed my mind.
My young nephew was very badly brought up. That's why I favoured a good upbringing. That's my sister's (step-sister's) boy. He was brought up entirely by my mother. He's 10. When he was small, he was never allowed to cry. And he's been very spoilt. He even answers back to my parents. I can't understand that. I said to my mother, "I jolly well won't give you mine to bring up."'

231

At this point, she digressed as follows:

> 'A little while ago, I had a bit of trouble. My nephew refused to do what
> I told him. I threatened him and he said, "I'll tell mummy". I said, "I'm
> not bothered about your mummy", and gave him a slap, not very hard.
> Two days later, he was naughty and rolled his eyes to frighten me. This
> led to trouble. My mother got angry and put us out. I've never liked this
> kid, this son of an unknown father. I've never forgiven my sister. I've
> never got on with her. She is hard and strict. I'm not like her. She was in
> love with a man who was getting divorced. She wanted a baby, and I said
> to her, "Think what you're doing, you're mad!" When she was pregnant
> she was even worse. Nobody dared tell me.'

She therefore had a rather prudish background: 'As for me, I was always
forward for my age and I was curious and asked questions. When I was
6, I found some contraceptives. I asked mummy what they were for. She
wouldn't ever tell me, she was embarrassed. So I found out from boys
and girls at school.'

On the whole, Mrs K thought that children should not be told things
except when they were old enough to understand the danger, for girls, of
getting pregnant: 'I'll do the same as my mother. I can realize that she
brought us up well.'

There was, therefore, considerable aggression against her mother,
rationalized in terms of the difference in the ways in which she and her
nephew were brought up.

Father. 'My father was even nicer than my mother. I used to blush when I
was face to face with my father. I didn't dare ask him questions. My father
was a widower, he had a son by a previous marriage, and my mother was a
divorcee and my elder sister is really a step-sister.'

Younger sister. Mrs K does not know the exact age of her younger sister,
but she is about 23. She gets on well with her: 'I can do what I like with her.'

Family background. Mrs K had been her father's favourite:

> 'I was always behind him, and, at table, on his knees. I had an accident
> with him on a bicycle. My mother didn't want him to take me. I was 5 at
> the time. My foot caught in the spokes. Fortunately, my father didn't
> brake or my foot would have been cut off altogether. As it was, it was
> only the tendons that kept it on.'

This epic episode left a small scar. 'It was my father who told me about it.
My mother was nearly out of her mind. "You've killed my daughter."' She
had her foot in plaster for two months:

'My father and my mother couldn't bear to come near me. The doctor had to come every day. He said to me, "If you cry, I'll give you an injection." My father never smacked me, except once when I nearly killed my sister. I didn't want to lend her my toy. I threw the tongs at her head. I was jealous of my sister, I didn't want her. When my mother was expecting her, I kept repeating, "I don't want it, I don't want it!" When my mother was feeding her, I tried to stop her, I didn't want her to touch the breast. I had to be taken away or I would have struck my sister. Afterwards, I got fond of her, I was crazy about her, nobody dared do anything to her while I was there.'

Jealousy did, however, persist, along with serious guilt feelings: 'Once, when we were playing, I twisted her arm. My mother said, "You've broken her arm, you did it deliberately", and slapped me.'

Older step-sister. 'She wouldn't take me out with her.' To return to the episode of her step-sister's pregnancy, Mrs K said that she was very angry with her for getting pregnant. Her sister however said, 'I'll never have a baby!' 'My mother had warned us so thoroughly. I thought she would have been angry with her, but she treated the matter as if it were quite normal. I asked her, "Is she going to have her baby adopted?" "No," said my mother, "I'm going to keep it." "And supposing I were to do the same thing?" And my mother began to cry, and I realized that that had upset her. I reassured her.'

Mrs K could not rationalize her behaviour here, and admitted that she did not know why she had teased her mother like that.

Older step-brother. 'He means a lot to me. He is everything to me. He is the very image of my father. He is good and kind. When he went off to the war, I cried.' He has been married for about thirteen years and has six children.

Her elder sister is now living with another man. Her younger sister has been married for two or three years. She is expecting her third child. Her first confinement was very difficult in its later stages. During her second confinement she did not feel anything.

Interests before marriage. 'I loved dancing tangos and waltzes. I wasn't interested in anything else.' She seems to have been very straight with boys. 'I could see right away if he was flighty. I didn't want to get married, I wanted to enjoy myself dancing first. As for sex, I hardly thought about it.'

First sexual relations. Mrs K associated: 'My sister is very cold, it's quite obvious. And she wears the trousers. I'm not like that. When I saw my husband, his eyes made me tingle like an electric shock. He asked me for it right away. I told him there was nothing doing.' Later, he promised himself that he would give her up if she kept refusing him for more than a certain time. 'I learned later that he had previously been in love with another woman who had denied him because she wasn't a virgin and she didn't want him to find out. He met her during the holidays and she told him she regretted it very much.'

Mrs K denied feeling in any way jealous. Her husband had wanted her to sleep with him without committing himself to marriage. He didn't want to get married immediately. She therefore had an affair which lasted six years, and it is difficult to get a clear picture of these six years: 'I was afraid of having a baby.'

The loss of her virginity was an event of great importance to her. 'In the end, I felt I had had enough. I said to him, "It's me or your father." These were the alternatives. My father-in-law didn't want us to have a baby right away. He didn't want to be called "grandfather". I simply fixed a limit and I said to my husband, "After I'm thirty, I'm having no more of it." And after that I never mentioned it to him again. It was he who finally made up his mind.'

Future. The interview returned to the question of the nursing period. Mrs K still did not know what she would do, but really wanted to give up work and not return to it.

Rapport was good. The patient was difficult to understand immediately and for that reason was allowed to carry on a somewhat trivial and occasionally rather incoherent conversation.

THIRD INTERVIEW WHEN OVER 8 MONTHS PREGNANT

Different psychologist.

Mrs K had not attended for her last appointments. She asked to be seen without having an appointment. She had just returned from holiday.

Pregnancy. She was a little more tired. Things were a little more difficult and the baby was moving a lot. 'But on the whole, I've had an easy pregnancy, except for the fact that at the beginning I was always asleep. I've never been ill.'

Mrs K had not been sleeping so well for some time. She had been waking up during the night to go to the toilet. She thought that the baby must have been pressing on her bladder. Sometimes she found it difficult to get back to sleep.

Mother's gynaecological history. The family situation was unchanged. Her mother was in Dordogne and would not be back for her confinement: 'She is tired. Perhaps it's her change of life. She is generally run-down.' She probably had her menopause about a year ago, but Mrs K was not sure. Mrs K had asked her mother about her confinement: 'She couldn't tell me what

234

happened. Everybody's different, that's what she told me. I asked her specially what it was like at the beginning. "If you take after me, you won't have much trouble with your confinement. Everything always went off very well." '

The second daughter, Mrs K's sister, had some trouble with her first child, but her other confinement and those of the elder sister had gone off very well.

Dreams. She had been dreaming. 'But it is a long time since I had a nightmare. At the beginning, I dreamed I saw my husband with another woman.'

Husband's attitude. She then explained that her husband had not wanted sexual relations since the fourth month because he was afraid. Currently, they were not having intercourse – 'even less', she said. When asked if she felt the lack of it, she said she did and she did not:

'From the fourth month I've felt less desire for it but all the same, there are times when you are near your husband, it's normal, isn't it, to have . . . My husband's afraid of doing me or the baby some harm. He has nightmares. He talks during the night, but he doesn't tell me about it. Sometimes he sits up in bed and shouts out, "Wait, wait, I'll see." In the morning he's forgotten what he dreamed and can't tell me.'

To start with she found her husband's attitude very irritating, and she thought that he was deceiving her, though he denied it. She went on:

'Now I have confidence, whether it's true or not. My friends thought it was funny (she had been talking about it), they think he must have a mistress, or else that he's abnormal . . . Anyway, it doesn't really bother me. And I don't particularly want it just now. And of course, my husband's a serious chap, he's not the kind to play around, unless I wasn't there at all (meaning, unless she was dead). That's some consolation.'

She would thus, in fact, appear still to be somewhat anxious on account of her husband's attitude.

She reported that she sometimes felt as if she could not breathe, as if she were suffocating, and she worried.

'During the holidays, I did a fair amount of travelling by car. My husband was afraid it might be bad for the baby. I was perfectly all right. I was almost lying down. My husband is very anxious. He's been afraid ever since the beginning of my pregnancy. First of all, he wouldn't believe it was true. If it's a girl, he wants to call her after his mother, Éliane, and he wants a girl . . . I would rather have a boy, but I don't really mind. I haven't yet thought of a boy's name, nor has my husband. I've looked up the almanac with my father-in-law. He hasn't any ideas for a boy's name either. I've nothing to complain about in my father-in-law. He never mentions his wife. He doesn't like talking about her. He must keep his memories. He was very fond of her.'

Confinement and superstitions. Mrs K stated:

'I'm not at all afraid. But sometimes, in the family, with its past history . . . My mother has frightened me a little. My sister saw a menagerie while she was expecting her son. She didn't dare say that she was afraid she might have a snake or a monkey for a child. I myself, when I was two months pregnant, turned and looked when I was passing a menagerie. I knew someone of my own age; she was frightened by a lizard and she touched her belly. Her child is supposed to have had a mark like a lizard on him.'

(This story had been told her by her mother and the friend was in fact a friend of her mother.) 'I don't want to do that, I'm so frightened!' ('To do that' was to touch her belly.)

She began to laugh and went back to her sister's confinement. 'My mother didn't want to be present at the birth. My sister insisted, saying she was going to die. My mother said to the doctor, "It's going to be a freak."' After the birth she was very relieved and the sister asked if there weren't any marks on her baby. 'Where I come from, these things are widely believed.'

Mrs K laughed when she told this story, but it seemed as if she really were not very sure. She added:

'Sometimes you do see people with marks. My sister has a strawberry mark on her neck. Perhaps my mother touched her neck when she was thinking of the strawberry she would have liked and couldn't have. My sister's little girl has a brown spot on her shoulder. Sometimes you see wine-coloured spots, and people say that these indicate a wish for wine which wasn't satisfied. I knew a chap before my husband, but he limped. I never noticed it, but my mother did, and she was afraid in case the children would be like that. I asked about it. He hadn't told me that he had a brother who was crippled from birth and couldn't walk. He must have had it from birth too. He had one leg shorter than the other (and she had broken with him for this reason).

My husband is basically a kid. He is very appealing. My father-in-law is very timid. He didn't dare tell me, but he let me find out that my mother-in-law had once had a miscarriage in getting off a train . . . And then, some time later, she had my husband.'

The father-in-law would have liked another child. Mrs K's husband was 19 or 20 when his mother died after a long illness. 'Yes, she caught a chill on the lungs during the war. She went to a friend's funeral on a bicycle.'

All this is rather vague and Mrs K was unaware of the numerous contradictions. When they were referred to, she was astonished, and said, 'Oh, I don't know, it's what I've heard, you know.'

Mrs K is a big woman, well-built and attractive in a buxom way, and healthy-looking. She spoke laughingly and with studied detachment about the country superstitions and about her husband's fears. But it seemed that behind this apparently calm and critical attitude there lay anxiety which she tried to deny, as it were, by magic.

MRS K'S CONFINEMENT

The observer made contact with Mrs K for the first time about 5.30 p.m. when the obstetrician came to see her because labour had not been advancing after the spontaneous rupture of the bag of waters in the morning. She had wakened rather wet, and said, 'I thought I had peed in the bed.' She refused to associate to this, and denied having ever been enuretic, but said, ambiguously, 'A child should be dry about the age of four or five.'

What at once struck the observer was the noise the woman made during her contractions. Although dilatation had not started, the impression given was of a woman in the transition stage, bearing down and restraining herself from doing so. She was making throaty noises and groaning like a woman with colic. She admitted in fact that at times she felt like bearing down, but that mostly it was the baby who seemed to want to force himself downwards. 'He's pushing, he's wanting to . . . ', and she indicated her lower abdomen and perineum. She assumed a tense expression, not so much of actual pain, as simply of effort, although hardly any bearing-down effort was then involved. Her respirations were spontaneously panting and deep, although she had received no such directions from the midwife: 'I do that in just the same way when I have my periods, which are very painful.'

She assumed a curious expression, shutting her eyes and making a forced grimace, as if she were trying not to vomit. She said that she was afraid of getting torn. The desire to bear down was 'like a ball wanting to come out; it's not like a bowel movement, but I can't tell you why. The midwife told me a little while ago that I was bearing down without realizing it, and since then I've been holding myself in.' She breathed like a bellows and that relieved her. 'It's my backside that hurts – I don't know whether its my backside or my kidneys.' In fact, she had acute pain in the sacral area. She now said, 'It's hurting in front down below; before, it was hurting higher up. It's hurting so much, I can't move.'

She seemed indeed to be pinned to the bed by her very considerable bulk. When contractions started, she said, 'Will it be long?' On the question of her refusal of preparation for childbirth, she said, 'My boss didn't want to give me the afternoon off to attend the course, and then I was away on holiday.' At the next contraction, she sought contact, holding out her hand: 'I can't stand any more.'

She had come to the hospital immediately after the spontaneous rupture of the bag of waters. 'My neighbour had explained all about it, that the rest followed, so I hurried. I was afraid it might happen on the way.' She must have filled up again during the journey. She continued to lose amniotic fluid intermittently at the hospital: 'When I was given my enema, I lost a lot.'

During another contraction, she said, 'He's pushing downwards.' She moaned. She established good contact, and spoke in a careful, deliberate way. She felt that the contractions were becoming stronger. She had had an injection the previous night, had slept and had woken up with pains. That same night, she was admitted to the labour ward. There had been no straightforward inception of the contractions. Several drugs were administered, including intravenous transfusion of posterior pituitary extract for a thickened cervix. She showed, therefore, delayed dilatation, a thickening of the cervix, and spasms.

As far as motor activity was concerned, she remained still except for her hands, as if she was unable to move any other part of her body. She grasped the observer's trousers, and then his hand. 'Now he's really pushing,' she said. She did not wish her husband to be present, but added, 'In one way, yes; in another way, no.' With some ambivalence, she said: 'In a way he would help me, but I think he would be disgusted with me afterwards.'

Paradoxically, she seemed to bear down less at this point. 'It's not a pretty sight when the baby comes out. It's the hardest part for me and for my husband. This morning I was worried. I felt that nothing was happening, that nothing was going to happen.'

She almost grabbed the observer's leg, which happened to be nearest to hand: 'I got the idea that the baby didn't want to come and that they would have to operate. I'm afraid of having an operation, I'm afraid of not waking up again. I would rather have a little boy – oh, I don't know, my husband wants a little girl.'

She grasped the observer's hand, and continued to hold it after the contraction. She squeezed it in time with her breathing. She remained still. When the observer said that he was going to call the midwife, she said, 'Don't leave me alone.'

The importance of the relationship at this time perhaps emphasizes the psychogenetic origin of the previous non-dilatation. A little earlier, when the doctor came, she was afraid, and was relieved that she did not need to have an operation.

6.45 p.m. 'Oh, how long it is!' She bore down harder. 'It's as if I wanted to go to the lavatory. It's uncomfortable because you're afraid of doing something.' It seemed as if dilatation had been speeded up because she was able to 'speak out', and thus to work off some of her fear. In the presence of the doctor and the midwife, her breathing was much more whimpering.

There was a contraction: 'Give me your hand.' The pain recurred: 'If it's painful, it finally gets you down; he's pushing.' Between contractions, her face was turned upwards, immobile, showing suffering with fortitude – an imposing mask. When she looked at the observer, she turned round slowly and gave him a bright, direct look. 'He's pushing. How I wish it was over.'

She had a nightmare at the end of her pregnancy: 'They were killing a man with an axe, and gashing him with blows of the axe to torture him. There was a woman who was having him killed; she was like a ghost, disappearing and reappearing at will.'

There was another contraction. In spite of her urge to bear down, she did not do so. She did not give the slightest sign of bearing down involuntarily. 'I hold my breath and keep from bearing down because that would hasten things – it's too soon.'

She was no longer whimpering as she breathed:

'It's passing! – In my dream it wasn't a film star, but a man I know, and then two men were arguing and I was preventing the little child from going to separate them because they had knives, and this wasn't the place to fight. I couldn't get along the corridor to go for help; the kid was smaller and could have gone, but he didn't want to. He was spattered with blood. – He's coming.'

7.10 p.m. She grasped the observer's hand more frequently. She wanted to change her position, made a few tentative movements, and finally appeared unable to move. She only raised her knees: 'I want to be free, to be able to get up and to walk. I'm so sore all over. I want to change my position.' She had an increasingly strong urge to bear down, accompanied by pains: 'I feel a bit squeamish.' She groaned. Her expression was quite different. 'I tell you, he's there, he's pushing.' She was panting a little. Her speech was most ambiguous at times.

7.20 p.m. She was now placed into position. At first she assumed a generally plaintive, downcast attitude which she had not previously shown – inhibition in the face of activity. The midwife was fascinated by the hairs which had resulted from the hormone treatment. The patient was difficult to get into position: 'I can't move, I'm worn out.' She seemed to regret her conversation with the observer. She seemed unable to get air. She groaned a little without bearing down, and was clearly prepared to 'hold it'. Suddenly, the contractions began to occur at intervals: 'He's surely going to come.'

239

On the second occasion she did not breathe, but bore down long and well. It was decided to use pressure: 'Just wait'; then, 'it's nearly over'.

The observer moved into the background. The contractions occurred at regular intervals. 'I'll wait; it will be Éliane or Michel.'

This woman gave the impression of holding herself in and retaining her baby. She gave the observer a nostalgic and rather lost look. She was bearing down very ineffectively, without breathing and apparently without determination.

7.35 p.m. Pressure was applied by the nurse. The observer encouraged her, saying, 'You can't go back.' She bore down a little better. After section of a strand of hymen, she really did not bear down any more; she seemed to have frozen.

A forceps delivery was finally avoided by the use of expression. She moved her toes while bearing down. She did not know whether she would be glad to see the baby, she was so exhausted. There was quite an energetic response by the staff – two nurses and two midwives, towards whom her attitude was one of withdrawal: 'I can't go on; wait a minute.'

Difficult issue at 7.45 p.m. She did not look, or show any interest. There was a discussion about the baby's clavicle. The patient seemed rather sulky: 'Little wretch, you hurt me; little rascal, you wouldn't come.'

She remained passive, her pain allayed. There was no sign of a relationship. She thought the actual birth would be more painful. She found it difficult to express herself. She was exhausted, overwhelmed by her obsessional tendencies. 'Alone, I couldn't have done it. It's funny to feel something there, like the first movements. I thought of nothing and no one . . . no one . . . just delivery.'

There was no sign of emotion, only relief on the mother's part. Michel weighed $8\frac{1}{2}$ lb. and was 21 inches long. The mother showed no reaction to the identity bracelet. Her face was expressionless. She lifted her eyes so that she would not see the placenta. 'I haven't been torn. I expected the worst. It was the fear of being torn, or of dying.' There was no haemorrhage and very speedy recovery. Expulsion had been rapid – twenty-five minutes, with pressure (otherwise, there would have been total inertia).

There was no immediate relationship to the child. Relations with others were permissive, and she was able finally to attain a degree of reassurance which was not, however, progressive. The baby was brought to her and she kissed his hands. 'Isn't he pretty!' she said in a whining voice, and asserted that she felt he was really hers.

SUMMARY

The case of this young woman is of particular interest. Although her experience as a woman had been difficult and guilt-laden, she refused to be prepared for childbirth. Faithful to her rural origin and farming background, in which birth is a 'natural' phenomenon, she preferred to let it retain its untouchable and quasi-magical quality, and rejected preparation which claimed to be scientific and undermined this mythical basis.

Her system of defences rested upon repudiation, denial, and isolation: these mechanisms served to protect her against her deep-lying anxieties with regard to childbirth.

Mrs K's score for negativity in her past history was 16, i.e. hardly above the mean (14) for women in this group. Her score of 15 for negativity during pregnancy was, however, considerably above the group mean (9·4).

Her total negativity score (31) was therefore especially loaded with present negativity, induced by the pregnancy crisis. The predominantly current nature of her negativity led one to hope for the kind of confinement which in fact she did have – a confinement scoring 25, i.e. rather poor but not disastrous. The stage of dilatation was one of inanition, obviously related to the patient's difficult and obsessional personality. On the other hand, the whole weight of the psychological pathology consequent upon the disorganizing impact of pregnancy did not entirely bear upon expulsion, and Mrs K recovered well during this stage and avoided a forceps delivery, partly thanks to a reassuring and permissive interpersonal relationship. This beneficial relationship seems to have operated in a similar way as that achieved by preparation, although quite clearly less coherently and effectively.

CONFINEMENT RECORD

07.00   Full-term pregnancy
        Foetal heart heard; head fixed
        Posterior lip of cervix flexible
        Membranes ruptured 24 hours previously: clear fluid
07.15   Second administration of spartine
        One cachet
07.45   15 cg. spartine
08.15   One cachet
08.45   15 cg. spartine
09.15   15 cg. spartine
09.30   Stretched cervix slightly dilated, foetal heart heard
10.45   Transfusion – 500 cc. glucose–serum
        Six mg. of 10 per cent methionate
        Five units of posterior pituitary extract
        1,000,000 units of Penicillin
11.40   Soft cervix dilated to one finger, foetal heart heard
        Head poorly flexed, with cephal-haematoma

241

12.00 Dilatation to about one finger
14.30 One finger; cervical band (anterior lip); foetal heart heard
Spasmalgine
17.00 One finger; cervical band (anterior lip)
17.40 Dilatation to two fingers; foetal heart heard
Spasmalgine
18.50 Almost full dilatation
Two units of posterior pituitary extract – coramine
Very rapid uterine contractions; foetal heart heard
19.50 Normal childbirth
Engagement of the head in the left occipito-posterior position
Delivery of the head in the occipito-posterior position
Birth of live boy, weighing 8 lb. 7 oz.
20.00 Complete normal delivery of the placenta, weighing 26 oz.
Transfusion – one bottle

BEHAVIOUR RECORD

First phase: taking up of cervix and dilatation to three fingers

    (a) *Psychological reaction* – patient quiet but anxious
    (b) *Muscular relaxation* – moderate

Second phase: from three fingers to full dilatation

    (a) *Psychological reaction* – patient nervous
    (b) *Muscular relaxation* – poor
    (c) Weak and intermittent groans
    Motor excitability
    Appearance of suffering

Third phase: expulsion

    (a) *Psychological reaction* – patient disciplined
    (b) *Expulsive efforts* – good
    (c) *Birth of the head* – easy, without episiotomy

Subjective assessment by patient

    Painful confinement

Comments

    Unprepared

Name: Mrs K   *Case Number:* X

Stage	Obstetrical index	Pain	Behaviour	Pain + Behaviour
Dilatation	2	3	4	7
Transition	1	3	4	7
Part total	3	6	8	14
Expulsion	2	3	3	6
Issue	1	2	3	5
Part total	3	5	6	11
Total over 4 stages	6	11	14	25

Activity : 2→3 at expulsion

Relations with staff: Quality 2
                                  Intensity 1

Relation to baby: Quality 2
                             Intensity 3

Preparation techniques:

	Use	*Effectiveness*
Breathing		
Relaxation		Patient unprepared
Bearing down		

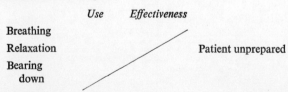

Explanatory comments:
  Pain difficult to assess except at stage of issue, which was described as practically painless.

  Behaviour tinged with a permanent malaise, and relationships with some degree of anxious tension.

NEGATIVITY GRID

Name: Mrs K

I. HISTORY	Childhood				Puberty-Adolescence				Adulthood			
	Mother	Father	Husband	Others	Mother	Father	Husband	Others	Mother	Father	Husband	Others
A Individual pathology												
(a) traumas											+	
(b) symptoms			+								+	
B Womanhood												
(a) gynaecological pathology											+*+*	
(b) inadequate information												
(c) negative incidents							+				++	
(d) difficulties concerning womanhood											++	
C Family background												
(a) traumas												
(b) pathology									+			
(c) interpersonal difficulties												+*
(d) disturbances in family environment											+	
D Social life												
(a) economic difficulties												
(b) difficulties over social adjust-												

II. PREGNANCY	Stage I	Stage II	Hospital adjustment
A General pathology			Unprepared
B Gynaecological-obstetrical pathology			
C Psychosomatic symptoms	+		
D Difficulties concerning womanhood and motherhood			
E Psychopathological symptoms			*Remarks*
(a) concerning woman	+	+	I = 16
(b) concerning baby		+	II = 15
(c) specific symptoms	+	+	Total = 31
F Character and behaviour disorders			

G Family troubles

	Stage I		Stage II	
	Mother	Family	Mother	Family
		++*		+
	Husband	Husband's family	Husband	Husband's family
	+*	+	+*	+

H Social and economic difficulties

Note: An asterisk denotes an item of special importance, which scores 2 points on the grid.

NOTES ON MRS K'S NEGATIVITY GRID

I. *Negativity in personal history*

A(a) col. 3 pleurisy
 (b) col. 1 recurrent tonsillitis
 (b) col. 3 hypertrichosis
B(a) col. 3 dysmenorrhoea, menstrual irregularities*
              amenorrhoea before marriage*
 (c) col. 2 broken engagement
 (c) col. 3 emotional break
              difficulty in getting married
 (d) col. 3 traumatic experience of first intercourse
              forceful and guilt-laden liaison
C(b) col. 3 mother: menopausal disorders
 (c) col. 3 difficulties with future in-laws*
 (d) col. 3 family taken over by father-in-law

II. *Negativity during pregnancy*

C   col. 1 pain in breasts, hypersomnia, vomiting
     col. 2 nausea, constipation, etc.
E(a) col. 2 fear of dying
 (b) col. 2 fear for baby
 (c) col. 2 anxiety dreams
F   col. 1 hypersensitivity, nervousness
G   col. 1 sister raped*
             sister's miscarriage
     col. 2 husband: cessation of sex life*
     cols. 1 husband: rejection of pregnancy, abortion proposed*
     & 2   husband's family: ambivalent dependence in rela-
             tion to father-in-law

Third Case-history

It was decided to present the case of Mrs D although it was not included in the sample on which the statistical analysis was based; it is in fact a case of forceps delivery. As indicated in Chapter 4, anaesthesia makes observations on such confinements very difficult to assess, and to compare with those on other cases. While it seemed necessary to omit these cases for methodological reasons, they are none the less of considerable clinical interest for an attempt to view the experience of childbirth in broad perspective. It therefore seems relevant here to present this case of forceps delivery, in which psychological factors play a most important part.

The case, furthermore, is one of a prepared woman, and provides an interesting illustration of the ineffectiveness of preparation when deep-lying inhibitions have to be dealt with.

The obstetrical and behavioural record of this case will be given, but there is no negativity grid or confinement grid, since the case was not included in the analysis.

MRS D

FIRST INTERVIEW WHEN 3 MONTHS PREGNANT

Mrs D is a woman who looks 40 years of age, and is in fact 38. She has heavy and rather coarse features. She is dark, with very dark eyes, and a warm, lively, and intelligent look. She was quietly dressed in casual clothes of good taste.

Information on civil status. Mrs D is 38 years of age, a secretary in a large firm. She lives opposite the hospital, and was married three years ago, at the age of 35.

Choice of hospital. Mrs D stated that the proximity of the hospital had of course influenced her choice, but that, in addition, she had heard of the good reputation of the maternity department.

Desire to be pregnant. Mrs D said spontaneously: 'I had a miscarriage in 1952.' This had been induced. She spoke about it without signs of guilt, and with a fair degree of objectivity. She said that she had induced the miscarriage herself with the aid of a probe. She explained:

'Of course, it was possibly through ignorance. I never thought of the risk I was taking. I know it's dangerous. But anyway, I did it because I had

246

made up my mind to do it. [*Q.*] Yes, my boy friend was much younger than me. Because of that, I didn't want to force him to marry me, so I preferred an abortion. And I did it without telling him. He was a student. I didn't want to have a student husband and a baby, to have to keep both husband and baby. I decided to have this miscarriage, knowing quite well what I was doing. Then I had a haemorrhage and they took me to hospital for a curettage.'

Her husband is 41 and is a works foreman. Mrs D explained that she had begun to despair of ever having a baby. She had been married for several years; the couple very much wanted a baby and Mrs D did not think she was sterile.

Current symptoms at the beginning of pregnancy. Mrs D considers the beginning of her pregnancy to have been bad because it had coincided with an attack of bronchitis. She was not immediately aware that she was pregnant, because, instead of amenorrhoea, there was a brief metrorrhagia which she had mistaken for a normal period. The pregnancy was discovered 'accidentally' in the course of a gynaecological examination for leucorrhoea which had become severe. This examination also took place at the time of her bronchitis.

The beginning of the pregnancy in fact went unnoticed since it coincided not only with an attack of bronchitis but also with a state of exhaustion induced, according to Mrs D, by the physical effort and mental strain involved in moving house.

She reported current nausea (she has never vomited) and an aversion to certain foods. There was also marked hypersomnia, the more remarkable since for several years Mrs D had not been sleeping well and had been taking sedatives regularly. Finally, she suffered from increasing constipation.

Psychologically, she felt that there had been little change. She described herself as always very nervous and as having had several attacks of tachycardia of nervous origin.

Feeding the baby. Mrs D had been nursed at her mother's breast until she was one year old. She would like to feed her own baby for at least two months – she is obliged to work. She explained that she would rather look after her baby and devote herself to it entirely, but that they have heavy debts because of their new flat, and that she will consequently have to work in order to increase their joint income.

Illness. Up to the age of 13, she had frequent bronchitis. She also had two attacks of broncho-pneumonia and, subsequently, a calcium deficiency. When she was 26 she had a tonsillectomy because of recurrent tonsillitis from the age of 20. Since this operation, she had been free from pharyngitis. At 27, she had diphtheria.

Motherhood and Personality

First menstruation. Mrs D had her first period at the age of 12. She said that she had never been warned about it by her mother, and that her mother 'always treated her like a child and never discussed the facts of life'. Mrs D said that when she was 17, her mother still talked of 'buying a little brother'. She remarked, without aggression, that she disapproved entirely of this kind of explanation, that 'it's a very bad principle, but the usual thing in the country', and that she did not 'hold it against her parents', but that she would certainly 'bring up her own child quite differently'. Her parents are farmers.

Father. Her father is 69. She described him as being in excellent health and never having been ill: 'I've never seen my father in bed.' He is a very thin man, very active, very jolly, and very full of life. He is still able to work like a young man. He looks after a holding and works hard. He rises very early in the morning and is extremely alert for his age.

Upbringing. Mrs D lived with her parents until she was 23, and up to that age apparently never went out by herself:

> 'Yes, I was very restricted. My parents were certainly very rigid. My father wouldn't hear of a girl going out alone. There was never anything doing. I never went out with a boy while I was living at home. Naturally I felt it, compared with my chums, who could go out with boys, and were much more free. I told that to my father, who replied, "When you're married, you can tell me what you like."'

Mrs D was not on close terms with her father who seemed, from her description, to have been a rather cold and authoritarian character who never beat his children but was feared by them. She remarked, 'One look petrified me.'

Mother. She described her mother as a very gentle woman, very much under her husband's authority. She is 67, and works with her husband. Mrs D explained that when she was little, if she did something silly, it was in her mother that she confided. She would never have told her father, she was so afraid of him, and she asked her mother not to tell him. Her mother therefore seems to have played the part of friend and accomplice, though very much under her husband's authority.

Siblings. She has a sister of 35 who is unmarried and lives in Paris. This sister lived with a man for many years, but he was killed in a car accident. She was very depressed after this accident but had now recovered. She is working and is independent and, according to Mrs D's description, more or less flourishing.

General course of Mrs D's life. Mrs D had taken a shorthand typist's course and had then remained at the farm, which was not at all to her liking. At

248

the age of 20, she spent a year as a secretary in a lawyer's office. She then went to the Electricity Board in the area, and began to think of leaving home and coming to Paris. She asked for a transfer to Paris without telling her parents and, when she got it, faced them with a *fait accompli*. She said that this caused less commotion than she had anticipated. They could appreciate the reasons for her leaving, since she represented it as an advancement in her career. In Paris she lived in a room by herself and, before long, got to know her boy friend, a youth younger than she, with whom she was very much in love, but whom she did not want to marry just because of the difference in age.

She described her first experience of sexual relations as very painful and never entirely satisfactory during this first affair. She had been very disillusioned by her first sexual experiences.

Mrs D gave the impression that she had had a fuller sex life than she indicated in this first interview, and we shall return to this later. She did, however, state that she had broken off this affair after her abortion and that, subsequently, she had always been very afraid of becoming pregnant: 'I didn't get any pleasure from it, and I was really terrified. I was horribly afraid of becoming pregnant again.'

She had an affair lasting three months with her husband before getting married. She reported that she had achieved very satisfactory sexual relations with him. Her marriage had not encountered any opposition from her parents. She said that they were very pleased and very fond of her husband:

'My husband is very nice with them, of course, but in any case they are very fond of him. They know that I am pregnant and they are looking forward impatiently to this child, who will be the first grandchild in the family, and also in my husband's family.'

Sex of the child. Both Mrs D and her husband want a boy.

Attitude to confinement. She said that she had not thought about it. She did not think she was particularly soft, and explained that she was not afraid of her confinement because she so desperately wanted the baby. She said that she was sensitive; other people's suffering affected her, but she thought that, as far as she herself was concerned, she was strong enough and tough enough. She wanted to have preparation. Her own doctor advised it and she therefore decided to do it. She believed that it consisted of techniques of breathing and relaxation, and that this would be very useful.

By the end of the first interview, this intelligent and already mature woman had established good rapport.

249

SECOND INTERVIEW WHEN 5 MONTHS PREGNANT

Same psychologist: the relatively easy but rather superficial relationship of the previous interview was re-established.

Current symptoms. Persistent hypersomnia, with considerable debility. 'Every evening when I come home from work, if it weren't for my husband, I would go straight to bed. I don't want to do anything, I don't want to go out, I'd just spend all my time in bed.'

In this connexion Mrs D referred again to the habit she had developed, since coming to Paris, of taking sedatives. She had tried a whole range of drugs and finally found one (phenobarbitone) that alone enabled her to sleep. At that time, she had suffered from nocturnal attacks of anxiety:

'I really had the blues, I was all tensed up; I worried about nothing. If I had several of the minor worries of everyday life, in the evening I was frightfully down in the dumps. Since I've been pregnant, I'm not like that at all, I've no more need of drugs.'

She is still very constipated. In this connexion, she reported that at the age of 15 she had had an intestinal infection consequent upon a long period of constipation.

Dreams. She said that at present she could not remember her dreams. She did not seem to dream any more.

Menstruation and illnesses. Mrs D had suffered from dysmenorrhoea until she was 23 or 24. Before this age she had sometimes vomited, and even fainted, during the first two days, and had regularly taken sedatives.

Mrs D then went into the question of her illnesses, and again referred to having had diphtheria when she was 27, going on to say:

'I have more confidence in hospitals than in nursing homes. I've great confidence in Paris hospitals, because I know that, previously, women used to die in childbirth, it was a serious matter, but now, they have everything in a hospital to save the mother and the baby, and the mortality is very considerably reduced.'

Fantasies. An attempt was made to find out more about these fantasies of death, and at this point Mrs D admitted that she sometimes thought about it and reasoned with herself, telling herself that nowadays there were no more accidents, and that she had not heard of any cases of women dying in childbirth. But it was something about which she had often thought, and was one of the first fantasies she had had concerning childbirth, since her pregnancy (guilt). She said that she was also very afraid of suffering and that the last stages of the confinement were always painful. She believed in preparation, but felt that any pretensions to painlessness where unjustified, 'because whatever you do, you can't give birth without suffering'.

Mother's gynaecological history. Mrs D's sister had been born prematurely at eight months. Her mother had a difficult confinement, requiring blood transfusions and, according to Mrs D, her life had actually been in danger. Mrs D added:

> 'Yes, but you understand, it was in the country, and they didn't have everything that was needed. They gave her transfusions, but they weren't able to get the blood immediately, and apparently my mother's life was in danger. Anyway, I know she suffered frightfully, because she always said, "If I got pregnant again, I would throw myself in the river."'

Future. For the immediate future, Mrs D indicated that she would soon be on holiday, and that she was going to her parents' home. She would be quite pleased to see her parents again; she was going with her husband. She said that she would go by train, because she found the car very tiring and it tended to give her pains in the stomach. In fact, she was terribly afraid of having a miscarriage: 'The last journey we made, we only went to the suburbs, with my husband, in our car, and I felt very tired. When we got home, I felt as if my ovaries were being torn out.'

Movements of baby. The baby had moved ten days previously:

> 'I was very surprised, it was rather exciting, I hadn't been expecting it to move; until it moved, I felt that it wasn't true, I didn't really think that I was pregnant. Now, I'm much more aware of it, and I'm very happy. I would like it to be moving all the time.'

Mrs D observed that the baby moved more when she herself moved, and said, 'I think perhaps I get in his way, he wouldn't move if I didn't.'

Baby's future. She had begun the layette, and had already made one vest. They had not quite decided on Christian names. If it is a boy, he will be called Philippe, Thierry, or Eric. She explained that she had suggested these names to her husband. She was asked how the couple arrived at decisions, and replied that she guided her husband a little without his noticing it, and generally managed to get her own way. In important matters, such as choosing a house or moving, she always decides and then persuades her husband to make the same choice. She felt most reassured by the proximity of the hospital – she lives just opposite – and commented: 'I tell myself, even if it happens during the night, I'll be there in time.' She is afraid that the baby might come too quickly, and is therefore reassured because the hospital is so close. She intends to go on working until her leave of absence. She wants to go back to work after the birth of the baby and she would try to get some local woman to look after the baby, since there is no crèche.

Husband's family. Mrs D's parents-in-law are both dead. Her father-in-law was stung on the head by a bee and died very suddenly, paralysed, in 1956. He lived in a village in the north. Her mother-in-law died at the age of 64: 'She died of a stroke.' Her husband was therefore 20 when his father died and 26 when his mother died. He was an only son. He had a younger sister who died when she was 3 or 4, and there is an elder sister. His mother was 40 when he was born. Mrs D described him as a very neurotic man who often lost his temper and was impulsive and lacking in self-control. She seemed to regard her husband as a child. She observed, 'It is most amusing to see how he believes that he's the boss.' He is very quick-tempered.

Previous and present sex life. She said that she had reduced the frequency of intercourse, though not cutting it out altogether, because it gave her abdominal pains, and further, she said, 'I just don't feel like it any more.'

She then reverted of her own accord to her emotional life before marriage, and spoke of her first affair before she had come to Paris. The boy had been a childhood friend, and she had had a rather ambiguous relationship with him. It had not been clear how things stood, and it was only shortly before they were to be married that she had the degrading experience of finding out that he had been having an affair with a woman of 44 by whom he had two children and who was threatening *her*. Her former fiancé in fact explained that he was giving her up to protect her. She said she had reacted very sharply to this, with a feeling of being shut in and cut off. It was against this background that she left home for Paris where she arrived, as she said, in a rather rebellious state. In fact, her first months in Paris were very unhappy, and for nearly six months she was in a truly depressive state, from which she recovered only gradually, thanks to her relations with people in the office.

She seems to have adoped at this time a personal strategy of overcompensation, invulnerability, and superficiality in regard to men, maintaining emotional distance. She was, she said, at the time regarded as cold and cynical. She said that she was afraid of falling in love, and did not want to do so, and at the same time she felt set against the idea of getting married. In fact, as she said, she was extremely lonely.

Her second affair with a student was extremely frustrating, but fairly well tolerated. She had apparently had two miscarriages, the first not too clearly, induced with quinine when her period had been ten days overdue; the second during the holidays, when her boy friend was away. She had herself induced the latter with a probe, which caused a serious haemorrhage, and she reached hospital with a very severe loss of blood. An emergency curettage was carried out. 'But it was better to have that than to be turned off by my family', she said. When asked whether they took contraceptive precautions, she said, 'Yes, he withdrew.'

She herself was completely uninformed, and in all her sexual relations she felt herself dominated and rather defiled. Sexually, her experience had also been a complete failure in the sense that she had never derived any pleasure from it, intercourse being, on the contrary, painful. After her miscarriage, she stopped seeing this student, and during the ensuing years had several affairs, all of a rather casual nature. By then, she said, she had given up the idea of getting married, but in fact she did basically retain a certain hope. She had been unwilling to give up the prospect of a home of her own – something like her parents' home, closely knit and secure, and she added that she had been living at odds with herself, and that she no longer knew where she was. She had been regarded as gay and frivolous, whereas in fact she was so kind and gentle, and in so much need of protection. Even now, she said, people still considered her as placid and secure, whereas basically she was extremely anxious.

It would appear that other people give her the impression of always misunderstanding her, while forcing her to assume a 'persona', a façade behind which she is unable to recognize herself.

She described an absolutely idyllic relationship with her husband, in whom she had complete confidence from the start. He had not been deceived by her façade and had clearly perceived her true nature. She claimed that she had experienced full orgasm after six months of intercourse, and that her sterility was related to a retroversion of the uterus. Basically, however, she herself attributed it to her miscarriages, as a kind of punishment, although her guilt had been projected onto the young man.

At the end of this second interview, it may be said that good rapport had been established, in spite of a show of control on her part. This woman appeared to have compensated relatively well, and to be fairly mature.

THIRD INTERVIEW WHEN 8 MONTHS PREGNANT

Different psychologist.

Symptoms. Mrs D reported:

> 'Until just recently I was extremely well, but since Friday I've had fits of dizziness. On Saturday morning, I had an attack. I felt fuzzy when I woke up in the morning. Then I had this fit of dizziness. And I've been feeling very tired for some time. But I've been sleeping well and I'm not constipated.'

253

Dreams. 'I can't remember,' she said, laughing. She thought. 'Oh, I dream about things that don't matter. My husband had to go to the dentist, and I dreamed that he telephoned and the dentist had gone to America. It's a funny kind of dream.'

Her husband had been having toothache since the holidays. He had a wisdom tooth which was hurting him. He had seen the dentist before going on holiday and had been told that the tooth would have to come out. He had put off having it out and was suffering intermittently. The dream that the dentist was in America would appear to have postponed the extraction to an even more distant date. It meant that the tooth could not be removed by that dentist. And Mrs D added, 'In my dream, I was annoyed that my husband should have to go to another dentist he didn't know.' She did not dream of the extraction. She does not usually dream. She has been dreaming only since her pregnancy; and she forgets her dreams very quickly.

Fantasies concerning the baby and the birth. 'Yes, I've been thinking about it since the sixth month. My sister was born without her left hand. She has a stump where her left hand should be. So I was afraid, afraid that my baby would be born like that.' She said that with a smile, and was clearly glad to have an opportunity to talk about it.

As far as her confinement is concerned, she said that she was not afraid at all. She was glad to be having preparation: 'It's a good thing, it reassures you', she said.

She does not want her husband to be present at the birth: 'I know that for him that would . . . The sight of blood upsets him, so he wouldn't be much help or comfort to me.' This was said with a smile.

Sex life. The couple have not had intercourse for two months: 'I've absolutely no desire for it, I don't get any pleasure from it.' Sexual relations actually became painful. She experienced no revulsion. Her husband is 'understanding': 'He doesn't talk about it. He seems to find it quite normal. Also, we thought at first that it might harm the baby. [*Q*.] No, I don't know how.'

Her husband is sure 'we'll have a fine baby; he isn't at all worried. My husband groans during the night. He groans a lot. But he's always been like that. I think he's dreaming, but he doesn't remember his dreams.'

Future. Mrs D's parents are coming for the confinement. They will stay at her place. She is very pleased that they are coming. 'I've been in Paris for ten years and they've never shown any desire to come. It needed this to bring them. They are coming to see their grandson. They are to stay for a fortnight. We'll take advantage of their visit and have the baby christened too.' Mrs D's sister is to be the godmother. The baby will be called Philippe if it is a boy and Isabelle if it is a girl. 'We would like a boy, but people say from the way I'm carrying it that it will be a girl.'

Mrs D is going to stop work on 16 August, but will return to work again after the leave of absence granted for the confinement. She has already put her name down at a crèche in the neighbourhood: 'It's a new crèche. There are only thirty babies, and I liked that. It's light and clean. If I do that, I'll have him every evening and Saturday and Sunday. With a nurse, you really lose too much.' Mrs D will feed her baby for the first two months: 'I'll feed him if I have enough milk. The doctor advised me to, because it gives children a good start.'

There is scarcely any financial problem in the household. The husband is earning about 1,800 francs per month and she is earning about 580 francs. They did, however, have to borrow money in order to buy the house in which they are living, and that is why Mrs D feels obliged to return to work after having her baby. She was asked whether they intended to have any more children. 'Oh, I've had so much trouble having the first, but even so, I wouldn't mind having two.' She felt less tense since becoming pregnant. She was very nervous before that. And also, her attitude to life is different: 'It's another link between us. My husband loves children. So do I, I've always liked children. Four years of marriage before this baby came. We were afraid we might not have any. And then, it came just when we had stopped expecting it.'

Mrs D's sister. Her disability has 'given her a complex'. She comes to see Mrs D every week. 'My husband is very nice with her. He has lost both his parents, and my family is more or less his own.' The sister works in an office.

'She is very different from me. She is irritable and quick-tempered. She has a headstrong and wilful nature, but she is very kind-hearted. She can't bear to see people in trouble. Physically, she is like my mother, whereas I am like my father. But my mother is gentle and self-effacing whereas my sister, it's her disability which has made her bitter and bad-tempered. For five or six years she lived with a man, but he was killed in a car accident. He was in some kind of business. It was during the war. He had escaped from Germany. He couldn't get married then. He would probably have married her after the war. Then he was killed . . . Everything that he had bought was in my sister's name. She is still in touch with her "mother-in-law" whom she still sees regularly, even today, and with whom she gets on well. She never had a child because she couldn't. She and her friend wanted children.'

Family background. Mrs D's mother was the youngest of five children, and lost her own mother when she was 3. She was brought up by an elder sister. Two of her sisters had no children. Her elder brother and another sister each had three children. Mrs D's parents were six years without a child, and then they had two daughters within an interval of eighteen months. Mrs D's sister was born a month premature. Her mother nearly died. For eight days she had had blood transfusions and had hung between life and death. Mrs D herself weighed 11lb. at birth. 'Childbirth wasn't as easy then as it is now', Mrs D remarked, 'but it went off all right.'

Her mother had had a very good pregnancy with her, but she had been constantly ill while carrying her sister. Mrs D's parents are an exemplary couple. They never argue, and have never been apart even for a single day. 'My mother is a saintly woman. She is very gentle.'

Her parents are very pleased about the coming birth. It will be their first grandchild, and they want a boy: 'They wanted a son and never had one. They were disappointed at having only daughters. Yes, they really wanted a boy when my sister was born.'

Pregnancy. Pregnancy has not changed her nature much: 'No, I'm not any more irritable than before. Perhaps I cry more easily, but I don't lose my temper. But I start to cry for the slightest thing. I'm very sensitive.'

At the end of the third interview, rapport was good. Mrs D was able to control acute anxiety over the possible difficulties involved in pregnancy and childbirth, the fear of having an abnormal child, and the fear of death.

MRS D'S CONFINEMENT

Mrs D had come into hospital on the previous day, and was in the prenatal ward. She had reoccupied the bed that she had had the previous month when it was thought that the date had been estimated wrongly and that the birth was imminent. She had been kept in a few days for observation. This time, she was all smiles and relaxed. She remarked, 'I hope I'll have it this time.'

She was in excellent form. She had had several sanguineous discharges, and had been hospitalized for that reason. The observer went back to see her again in the afternoon. She started off again spontaneously:

'It's awful with me. It's always the same. If I'm going anywhere, I set off very early. I'm never late. If I'm doing anything, I'm generally very slow about it. When I begin something, for example my baby's layette, it's the same thing. When I begin a vest, it takes ever so long. I'm a slow worker. I prepare well in advance for anything. I've a horror of anything hasty. What's done in a hurry seems to be badly done.'

When she was visited, the obstetrical team thought that the baby would be born that night. At this point, the psychiatrist informed the midwife of the psychological prognosis of a difficult confinement. The following day, Mrs D was still not in labour. The observer saw her in the prenatal ward. She was beginning to get restless and felt several mild contractions. During the

256

afternoon she went into the labour ward, and at this point observation of her confinement really started.

She had not slept the previous night, and said that this morning she was tired. Labour had now started. She had very frequent contractions and was beginning to complain of lumbar pains.

The observer saw her again at midday. Labour was progressing rapidly. Her contractions were quite frequent; she felt them in the back. She was breathing well. Her lips were dry. She was still calm. When the observer approached her, she seemed to be glad of his presence and reassured by it. She was between three and four fingers dilated and had pains in the back and severe lumbar pains. The observer sat down near her. Whenever she felt a contraction, she stroked her belly and said, 'It's not so bad when I rub my tummy.' The observer stayed a fairly long time alone with her. The midwife examined her. Rapport with the midwife was good. She felt lumbar pains only during contractions. Between contractions she talked, and said that she wanted a little boy, that she hoped for Philippe, that she wished it was over and that she was beginning to feel that she had had enough of it. But her overt behaviour was calm. She remained well relaxed and did her breathing well.

At the beginning of each contraction, she massaged her lower belly and gave a little gasping breath. The midwife took up her position beside her and encouraged her: 'It's going nicely . . .'

She began to feel the desire to bear down. 'He's pushing,' she stated, a little frightened. The midwife said, 'You're hoping for a boy, but if it's a girl, what will you call her?'

'If it's a girl, she'll be called Christiane, but I would rather it was Philippe.'

She was still relaxed, still breathing well and doing her relaxation exercises effectively. But immediately after her first impulse to bear down, a change in behaviour appeared. She got worked up and said, 'I can't go on, I can't go on bearing down, I'm so tired.' She said this quite loudly. At one point, the observer was talking to the midwife about administrative matters. Mrs D felt that she was being abandoned and felt for and caught hold of the observer's hand, which was quite a distance from her. She whimpered and said, 'I can't go on like this.' The observer said, 'We won't leave you.'

At this point, the midwife examined her again: 'There's still a little bit to go. You're not quite fully dilated. But the head is descending. Soon it will be time for you to bear down.' She said, 'Oh, I can't, I won't be able to bear down.' She clenched her hands and held back from bearing down. The midwife encouraged her but she answered, 'I won't be able to bear down, I tell you I can't bear down, I feel so awful.' She was given another injection. She tensed up and the midwife said in a mildly peremptory tone, 'You're getting

257

upset, there's no need for that. You've been very calm so far. Now you've got to bear down.'

During one contraction, she became very agitated. She moved her legs from side to side. The midwife explained that bearing down was the last stage, that she must be active, and that one is never completely exhausted. Mrs D took refuge in exhaustion: 'I can't, I tell you I can't, I just can't.' And she started a mournful recitation, in a whimpering voice, 'My tummy, my back, my buttocks.'

The midwife looked at her and told her to think of her baby. She smiled and relaxed, but at the next contraction she showed the outward signs of great suffering. She became tense and restless. Since the first impulse to bear down there had been a complete change in her behaviour. Whereas she had been calm and well controlled, she was now in a state where she suffered pain in a passive way, externalized it, became agitated, lost control, and whimpered like a child. She stroked herself and said, 'It doesn't stop any more, I can't do any more, it's pushing and hurting me.' She clenched her hands. The midwife said, 'You must bear down. Push against my finger.' She began bearing down, but did so ineffectively. She pushed from the chest, and not at all from below. Several feeble attempts at expulsion were attempted, and at the same time her anxiety increased. She became agitated and said, 'I can't, I won't manage, I can't.'

The midwives started to encourage her vigorously. The tension in the atmosphere mounted, charged with aggressiveness towards her: 'You've jolly well got to push, do as if you were on the lavatory . . . I'll help you,' and the midwife began to take up her position for expression, which terrified Mrs D. 'No, I can't, I can't.' The midwife said, 'This is it. You can't go back. You've got to produce your baby.' At this point, contractions ceased entirely. She would no longer bear down. Everyone stopped. They said, 'Come on, we're waiting for you.' She began, in a supplicating tone, 'Let me have the forceps, I tell you I can't. You're not in my place, you don't know what it's like. I can't, give me the forceps. I've been like this for two days, I haven't slept, I can't go on.' Unfortunately, Mrs D heard the team talking about forceps: 'Yes, yes, I want the forceps. You've got to, you can't let me go on like this.' The midwives encouraged her and scolded her, with some aggressiveness: 'You can't because you won't try.' And Mrs D retreated further and further into her blank refusal: 'No, I can't, I can't do any more.'

It should be noted that this woman was tired, but she spoke in a strong voice and refused *with energy* to bear down with her baby. Another attempt was made to apply pressure. The midwife took up her position, pushed on her belly, and at this point Mrs D turned and tried to bite her. The midwife telephoned to the house-surgeon who came immediately, asked no questions, donned his white coat, and put Mrs D to sleep. The mask had already been got ready. While the mask was being prepared and the house-surgeon called, the midwife had made one last attempt to get Mrs D to bear down, but it was too late. The labour ward was in a commotion and the midwives and nurses were bustling about.

Mrs D was anaesthetized very easily. She did not become excited, she really seemed to have been waiting to be put to sleep. The house-surgeon made a very easy forceps delivery, with episiotomy. The baby was at the vulva. He was a very big baby, a fine boy of $9\frac{1}{2}$ lb.

The observer waited until Mrs D recovered consciousness. As soon as she opened her eyes, the midwife asked her what had happened. She replied, 'I can't remember where I'd got to.' They said, 'How far have you got?' She said, 'My baby?', whereupon the observer replied, 'You've got a fine boy.' The obstetrical team had earned the beaming smile of this delighted woman. Immediately, she thought of herself again, and said, 'My goodness, how awful it was. I just couldn't do any more, you know, it wasn't my fault.' She was reassured: 'No, it's never anybody's fault, it wasn't your fault.' The observer told her that he would discuss it with her again, adopting an attitude of qualified approval towards her, because he felt that she regarded him as making common cause with the midwives and nurses, and possibly holding it against her for not bearing down.

There was an excellent immediate relation to the baby, which she desperately wanted, while at the same time fearing that she might never have it.

SUMMARY

Mrs D was exceptional in being primiparous at the age of 38. She had been brought up in the country by farming parents, in an atmosphere of paternal authoritarianism. Her life had been marked by: chronic constipation; serious respiratory disorders; two voluntary and guilt-laden miscarriages; the knowledge that her mother's life had been in danger when her sister was born prematurely with a stump instead of a left hand, and that her mother had had a difficult confinement when she herself was born late and very big; and previous emotional and sexual failure, which meant that her earliest sex life as a woman was unsatisfactory.

The result of these features was a deep-lying insecurity which found physical expression, but was partly offset by her intense desire to have a child, and by a good relationship with her husband. This explains why Mrs D had a relatively easy and sometimes euphoric pregnancy.

The reading of her case-history, however, indicates very high negativity, according to the criteria laid down in Chapter 5, mainly in the area of womanhood. It was precisely this cluster of pathological factors connected with her womanhood that we foresaw would be difficult to neutralize by a rather superficial collective form of preparation, such as is currently provided by hospitals. It would seem reasonable to suppose that only psychotherapy aimed at the pathological nexus would have helped this intelligent young woman to overcome the fear of being torn apart, which overwhelmed and inhibited her at the moment of issue, and caused her to demand anaesthesia as the only possible refuge.

It would seem that this burden of anxiety, together with the poor conditions in the labour ward (where tired midwives were unable to withstand the woman's anxiety and her reactive aggressiveness), led to the need for forceps, which can therefore be regarded as partly psychogenic. It is, however, noteworthy, that the baby was a big one.

CONFINEMENT RECORD

09.00 Full-term pregnancy
       Cephalic presentation fixed in high position
       Back to the left; foetal heart heard
       Posterior lip of cervix closed; membranes intact
10.00 Posterior lip of cervix flexible

Next day
09.00   Cervix almost completely taken up; flexible
        Foetal heart heard; few uterine contractions
10.15   Cervix easily admits a finger-tip; foetal heart heard
11.00   15 cg. spartine
11.30   15 cg. spartine
11.45   Cervix dilated to two fingers; foetal heart heard
13.00   Three fingers dilatation, rather thickened anteriorly
        Artificial rupture of the membranes: clear fluid
        10 cc. of 20 per cent methionate, intravenously
14.15   Dilatation between three and four fingers; foetal heart heard
15.15   Full dilatation
        Head at the vulva
        Expulsive efforts
15.30   Poor expulsive efforts
        Two units of posterior pituitary extract
15.40   Application of Gilles forceps after preventive episiotomy, for
        arrest of presentation (poor expulsive efforts)
        Engagement of head in left occipito–anterior position
        Rotation and delivery in occipito–posterior position
        Birth of live boy, crying normally, and weighing 9 lb. 10 oz.
15.45   Manual removal of placenta weighing 28 oz.

260

15.50   Repair of the episiotomy with catgut and six clips
General anaesthesia: Schleich
Penicillin, streptomycin

PREPARATION RECORD

First phase: taking up of cervix and dilatation to three fingers

    (a) *Psychological reaction* – patient calm, relaxed
    (b) *Muscular relaxation* – average

Second phase: from three fingers to full dilatation

    (a) *Psychological reaction* – patient calm
    (b) *Muscular relaxation* – average
    (c) *Breathing* – average

Third phase: expulsion

    (a) *Psychological reaction* – patient undisciplined, passive
    (b) *Expulsive efforts* – poor
    (c) *Birth of the head* – preventive episiotomy; forceps

Subjective assessment by the patient

    Severe lumbar pains

Comments

    Duration of labour – 5 hours; expulsion – 20 minutes of poor efforts
    Behaviour quite good during dilatation, but refusal to bear down

G. GAYLE STEPHENS, M.D.
3232 East Pine
Wichita, Kansas   67208

Critical Review of the Literature on the Psychology of Pregnancy and Childbirth and on Preparation for Childbirth

The aim of this appendix is to give an account of a number of recent publications. Some have already been referred to in the present work, to which they are directly relevant in view of the studies which they report. Here they will be reconsidered from an analytical and critical, and therefore wider and more general, point of view. Other studies have not received previous mention because they were not relevant to the main purpose of our research, but they should not be ignored since they represent appreciable contributions to the general literature on the subject.

In an attempt to make this critical review less tedious and more useful, the studies involved have been grouped under four headings:

I General psychological studies of pregnancy.

II Attempts to develop classifications of pregnant women; to establish relationships between personality, pregnancy, and confinement; and to predict the quality of confinements.

III Studies in which emphasis is laid on certain special factors such as rejection and acceptance of the baby; mother-child relations, etc..

IV Studies dealing with current problems; recent studies concerning preparation for childbirth.

Under each of these headings, a brief indication will be given of the particular frame of reference within which the problems are posed and considered: the ethnocultural or sociocultural approach, psychologically oriented obstetrics, experimental or clinical psychology, psychoanalysis.

Such a double classification by content and by level, although it may appear to some extent artificial and forced, is necessary in the interests of clarity and intelligibility, which are not always easy to achieve in a complex and rapidly developing field. Some writers, for instance, classify the women according to nervous type, or the results of projective tests, or personality data in general; others according to the degree of 'maturity', which is assessed after and on the basis of the pregnancy itself. Some regard anxiety as a factor operating in an overt manner; others endeavour to take account of deep-lying anxiety. Some see preparation for childbirth as the learning of a set of physical techniques, others as a form of mental hygiene, and others again regard it as a kind of 'emotional orthopaedics'. This indicates how far the level at which the psychological factors involved are presumed to act affects the level and interest of the respective studies themselves, and how it influences the assessment of these factors made by a given research worker.

I. PSYCHOLOGICAL STUDIES OF PREGNANCY

A number of studies carried out by obstetricians concerned with their patients are, in effect, descriptions of their experiences as practitioners, or accounts of their observations of pregnant women.

Some list the symptoms occurring during pregnancy, their frequency, severity, and development, providing a kind of indexed catalogue, as, for example, Harries and Hughes (67).

These lists are of interest when compared with other lists compiled for other cultures. Thus, in connexion with vomiting, various investigations have indicated that this symptom is a kind of 'cultural infection' (99). Such studies, still in their infancy, show the importance of the development of cross-cultural research. This interest is also shown in the growth of a specialized review, founded in Canada in 1956, concerned with relations between culture and mental health (147).

Other writers, in an attempt to adjust and improve their medical approach, analyse the most frequent difficulties of pregnancy and conclude in favour of a more enlightened attitude which would be more favourable to pregnant women, whether during prenatal consultations, or during the progress of the confinement in the labour ward, or during the patient's stay in the maternity department – see, for example, Chapman (26). Several articles lay down the elements of a real mental hygiene of pregnancy, confinement, and puerperium (cf. Lawton and Sisko, 95; Strauss, 145; and Fries, 63).

Some studies emphasize the pre-existence and predominance of the ethnic or cultural context in the experience, history, and meaning of the pregnancy, as well as in the progress of the confinement. Every society provides its pregnant women with 'models' of pregnancy, confinement, birth, and mother-child relations. The successful adjustment of the young woman to these cultural 'models' means a good pregnancy and a good confinement for her in her cultural context. This idea was developed by Margaret Mead and Niles Newton in their contribution to the First International Congress of Psychosomatic Medicine and Childbirth (106).

Mead and Newton give us a profitable lesson in cultural variation and relativity. Thus our own conception of a good confinement is not that of other peoples, and our experience of pain is different from theirs, both in respect of the feelings involved and in respect of its significance. (These ideas have been further developed and fully documented by Newton in a recent article (116).) Mead and Newton appear to return, however, after their accounts of childbirth, to the idea of a limit determined by what is biologically normal and physiologically natural. On the one hand, they write: 'there is no such thing as natural childbirth if we mean by that term physiological childbirth without any cultural overlays. Patterned behaviour always exists around the event of birth in human beings', but nevertheless they conclude: 'People who work with parturient women must accept patterning as inevitable. The only thing that can be done is to foster selectively those patterns that seem more in tune with *physiological cues*[1] and play down those patterns that are likely to interfere with smooth physiological functioning' (p. 54).

May there not be, in addition to patterning of birth, bodily, biological, and physiological patterning? May not biological and physiological functioning themselves be culturally influenced in some degree? This sort of question raises basic problems posed by the anthropological and cultural points of view. These problems have recently been considered by Brisset (20), who takes up the themes analysed in considerable detail by Dufrenne in his thesis (51).

Other writers, such as Rosengren, emphasize the importance within a given society – their own – of the environment, of the social status of the woman, and of the view of pregnancy as an illness, for determining the behaviour of women during pregnancy or childbirth. In fact, these writers play, for specific social groups, an anthropologist's role comparable in some ways with that of Margaret Mead.

In a first article, Rosengren shows that the tendency of the woman to view pregnancy as an illness is related to social instability and dissatisfaction with living conditions (141). In a later and more central article (142), he shows that there is a relationship between, on the one hand, duration and difficulty of the confinement, and, on the other, the indisposition of the mother who views her pregnancy as an illness, together with the physician's prognosis for the pregnancy and confinement, these two last factors interacting with one another.

These studies are of interest because they bring out the inevitable and very important process of previous social conditioning; but they do not explain why pregnancy should be regarded and experienced as an illness. Valabrega in his recent book (148) examines the equation of pregnancy with illness from a psychoanalytic point of view. He writes: 'The whole process from the beginning of pregnancy until confinement develops almost like a series of illnesses, or even one single long illness. Pregnancy is an illness from which

---

[1] Present authors' italics.

the woman is only *delivered* by her confinement, and this process of liberation is itself another illness which has to be gone through in order to be cured of the first. In every case, therefore, it is only *after* going through such a series of illnesses – and according to the pattern imposed by the initiation rite or illness – that the woman is able to adjust to a new stage by a redirection of her libidinal economy' (p. 173).

Valabrega further emphasizes the vital importance of the therapeutic relationship between the pregnant woman and the obstetrician both for the progress of the pregnancy and the confinement, and for the woman's psychological structure: 'It might be said that as soon as pregnancy is confirmed, the woman enters into a therapeutic relationship which continues for months and only comes to an end after the confinement, or even later. This is why one can observe in the relations of the woman with her gynae-cologist the whole range of patient-behaviour and all the elements involved in the therapeutic relationship, especially the more regressive ones, in a particular light' (ibid.).

Valabrega goes on to show how methods of preparation reduce the illness element in parturition by breaking the association of childbirth with illness (i.e. the equating of woman with patient), and observes that these methods are effective only because 'a prolonged psychotherapeutic relationship is established' (p. 174), which implies that 'the illness is indeed treated as such, but by other means and in another place. It is "displaced forward", and in this way becomes amenable to preventive treatment; what is an illness can only be dealt with by therapy' (ibid.). This represents a very clear position in the debate referred to in Chapter 1, concerning the history and develop-ment of preparation for childbirth, 'psychotherapy or psychoprophylaxis'.

Niles Newton (114) studies the emotions involved in pregnancy while keeping at the level of the social expression of psychological facts. She defines these emotions as those that 'every feeling woman may have towards every aspect of the feminine physical part she plays' (p. 2), and classifies them by external criteria into feelings about menstruation, pregnancy, childbirth, breast-feeding, infant care, the wish to be a man, sexual relations, etc. She wishes to find out whether there are any connexions between these 'maternal emotions' and 'other physical, psychological and social phenomena' (for example, between the wish to be a man and the wish to have a boy or the inability to nurse a baby), and demonstrates the existence of relationships of this kind.

In a later article (115) she considers, under the heading 'Emotions of pregnancy', all the relevant current literature. This article constitutes an extremely valuable analytical and critical bibliographical review. Newton illustrates the increasing interest in pregnant women, examines the emotional problems of pregnancy and childbirth from an objective scientific point of view, and summarizes present-day findings and hypotheses. In this very valuable work there is no attempt to get inside these emotions, to place them in context or to understand them; but their existence is recognized and they have become the object of systematic and statistical investigations.

The importance of the work of Bibring and her colleagues (13, 14, 15) lies in their attempt to get inside the problems of pregnancy and explain them. We are indebted to Bibring for the idea, which has fortunately become quite generally accepted, of pregnancy as a physiological and psychological crisis, that is, first of all, as a state in which the ordinary psychological and psychiatric criteria of normal and abnormal are inapplicable. Such acute and frequent revivals of former conflicts cannot be viewed in terms of the usual standards. A crisis includes stages of both regression and progression, and the balance between regression and progression is determined by the woman's personality development when she becomes pregnant – by her structures, defences, ego strength, and capacity for adjustment, i.e. by a complex of factors bound up with her life-history and expressing her condition in general. This implies the specific focusing on pregnancy of the searchlight already provided by the valuable earlier work of Helene Deutsch and Freud, especially their joint chapter on 'The psychology of women in relation to the function of reproduction' (45), which takes its place among Freud's numerous writings on female sexuality (57, 59, 60), and Helene Deutsch's paper, 'The significance of masochism in the mental life of women' (43), all of which contribute to the basis of Deutsch's main work, *The Psychology of Women* (44). The points of view of Deutsch and Bibring provide a firm basis for the more serious present-day work on pregnancy, on the crisis of motherhood, and on the emergence of the maternal role (cf. below the work of Racamier on this subject).

The basic method of investigating and reporting on pregnant women is simply to observe and describe them. The observation of an individual case, the tracing of a history back to its origins, the rediscovery of the conflicts, and the mapping of its development make a unique contribution, not only because there can be no substitute for clinical knowledge, but also because such a procedure reveals data from which extrapolations and generalizations may possibly be made. Unfortunately – and contrary to what one might expect – there are very few exhaustive and carefully carried out observational studies of pregnancy and childbirth. This may be in part due to the fact that this kind of study represents a new departure and calls for a high degree of perspicacity and determination, as well as a methodology capable of reconciling the practical difficulties involved, the requirements of objectivity, and the need to respect the subject's own personal feelings.

Here, we may refer to the works of Hernon Quijada (70) and Fox (56). The latter reports in detail the case of a woman who experienced a period of acute anxiety during the seventh month of her pregnancy, and gives an account of her psychoanalysis.

From the psychosomatic and psychoanalytical points of view, the following works are of particular interest: Menninger (108); Parks (122), who investigates ambivalence as a factor producing anxiety; Reynolds (140); and Pleshette *et al.* (129). All these studies attempt to assess the importance, repercussions, and somatic effects of emotional conflicts during pregnancy and childbirth.

With regard to the more specific study of pain, of its manifestations and significance, frequent attempts at quantification and scaling have been made (cf. Chapter 3) in France and elsewhere, in respect of both prepared and unprepared childbirth – unfortunately before any sufficiently long-term systematic analysis had been undertaken of the incomparable fund of data provided by the objective observation and description of the behaviour of women in pain. Here, Kammerer's paper (81) presented to the Congress of the Société française de Psychoprophylaxie obstétricale at Strasbourg (23) is relevant. Kammerer advocated the systematic collection of all the fantasies of pregnancy and childbirth with a view to obtaining as complete a picture as possible of the fantasy life that underlies everyday life, gives it its true meaning, and provides a key to its understanding. He thinks that only on this basis can working hypotheses be reliably formulated as to the scope and significance of pregnancy and childbirth, and also of suffering. It should, however, be noted that a study of this kind, however essentially desirable, may nevertheless sometimes be difficult to realize in practice. Some forms of preparation actively encourage the women not only to practise the techniques they have learned, but also to exercise an increasing degree of behavioural and emotional control, and there remains hardly any room for the expression of fantasies within such an institutional, practical, and mental framework. It is only within the context of more flexible and permissive modes of preparation that such material can find expression.

II. CLASSIFICATION OF PREGNANT WOMEN AND CONFINEMENTS, AND PREDICTABILITY OF CONFINEMENTS

As has been indicated above, there are not a few difficulties inherent in the collection of controlled observations, and these difficulties are greatly increased when, in an attempt to impose a framework that will enable the phenomena observed to be quantified or compared, investigators set up systems of classification, i.e. select their data according to one or more criteria.

1. There is a whole series of studies which classify pregnant women in terms of factors antecedent to the pregnancy or not directly relevant to it, and

unrelated to the specific problems of this critical period. These need be mentioned only briefly here, this subject having been discussed in detail in Chapter 3, to which the reader is referred. The various types of classification used are as follows:

(a) classification according to nervous type (79, 125);

(b) classification in terms of Berger's or Le Senne's characterology (96);

(c) classification in classical psychiatric terms (problem of normality and abnormality; studies of disorders as hysterical, paranoid, phobic, etc.);

(d) degree of overall adjustment achieved, and study of the possibilities of adjustment, with reference to family life, social, professional, or sexual life, etc. (the norm in this case is 'satisfactoriness' in terms of sociocultural requirements, or a good 'adjustment score');

(e) classification based upon principles derived from psychoanalysis: for example, in terms of progression and regression, or of the intensification or breakdown of defences, etc. (cf. Deutsch, Bibring);

(f) classification based upon performance on various tests, such as the MMPI (Hooke and Marks, 71), the TAT (Davids and De Vault, 40), etc.

Of these, (a) and (b), although interesting, seem to be too far removed from the essential data of pregnancy to be of real value for the psychology of pregnant women and the understanding of confinements. The others may appear more justifiable without being really relevant, and in fact are inadequate for the same reason – the uniqueness of pregnancy. The changes in thresholds, the shifts in perspective, and the more or less serious disturbances, interspersed with more frequent and rapid adjustments, require appropriate criteria which will facilitate the construction of a flexible and comprehensive scale that takes proper account of the problems of pregnancy and the overall pattern of this critical period.

2. In an attempt to avoid these pitfalls, some writers have devised their own scales for assessing pregnant women, in accordance with the orientation of their own research. Some systems have been established on the basis of assumptions derived from previous clinical experience and after a pilot study conducted with a small number of cases. They have the advantage of taking into account both the actual data yielded by a controlled study, and what is already known about the psychology of women and mothers to be, and about its relevance to the development of their children. Thus, in Pavenstedt's work (123, 124), the basic hypothesis is that the degree of maturity or immaturity of the mothers, as estimated during pregnancy, influences the development and maturation of their children. The pregnant

women in her sample were accordingly divided into three groups of high, medium, and low maturity in terms of their effective functioning and adjustment to general social and psychological requirements. The children were studied at various ages, and any behaviour disorders, assessed clinically, were related to the degree of immaturity of their mothers. 'Maturity' is an interesting criterion here, because it is central, covering the whole process of development as a woman and also taking account of the reorientation consequent on pregnancy. There is, however, some difficulty over the concepts of maturity and immaturity, which seem to be a little uncertain. Since they are used in such a way that they reflect mainly social adjustment, they leave little room for unusual solutions, or for those forms of regression that may in fact be followed by real progression, which occur frequently in pregnancy.

Another group of American workers, Davids, De Vault, and Talmadge (41, 42), hypothesize that anxiety is the key factor in pregnancy, and that it should be useful to relate it to the progress of the confinement. The hypothesis is not a new one, and other more clinical and less systematized investigations, such as that of Klein, Potter, and Dyk (83), have found support for it. In the work of Davids *et al.* anxiety was assessed at different points during pregnancy by the Taylor Manifest Anxiety Scale. When these scores were related to evaluations of the confinements, the hypothesis that highly anxious women would have worse confinements than other women was confirmed. This study includes an interesting bibliography on the attempts that have been made to quantify anxiety.

A difficulty already arises in connexion with the evaluation or classification of confinements. Although it is relatively easy to define a good confinement in obstetrical terms, it is less clear what constitutes a good confinement from a psychological point of view. Is it a painless confinement, a confinement free from anxiety (manifest or deep-lying), or a confinement that may be both painful and anxiety-laden yet represents a definite step forward in the mother's life (cf. Chapter 3, pp. 49-50)? Davids *et al.* used the simplest kind of criterion, an obstetrical evaluation based on both duration and difficulty of confinement.

A more serious difficulty concerns the nature of anxiety during pregnancy, and what the Taylor Scale really measures, in particular whether it reflects the amount of anxiety existing at the different stages of pregnancy, or the extent to which such anxiety is or is not expressed, i.e. the way in which the woman handles it, defends herself against it, and reacts to it. In the course of their research the present writers used the same criterion as Davids and his colleagues, the Taylor Scale, applying it to two samples of pregnant women: the women in one group were being prepared for childbirth, whereas those in the other group had refused preparation. The more anxious

269

women were to be found in the preparation group; the less anxious women refused preparation but had the poorest confinements. The women in the preparation group, who were perhaps more anxious to start with, indicated, by wanting preparation, that they were willing to accept reassurance or actually sought it. Several different kinds and levels of anxiety are therefore involved (cf. Chapter 7), and in work like that of Davids *et al.* this key notion of anxiety seems to be insufficiently analysed and perhaps inadequately measured by the Taylor Scale.

It would appear to be of great interest and value to assemble a wide range of clinical observations which would enable levels and aspects of anxiety to be established in advance through verbalizations, symptoms, dreams, and fantasies, with a view to demonstrating relationships between anxiety and duration and painfulness of confinement. Brown considers this question in an article (22) in which he attempts to elucidate the relations between anxiety and the psychosomatic disorders of pregnancy. After studying 150 pregnant women, using a number of different variables (two questionnaires, Taylor Scale, MMPI, extraversion, etc.), Brown concludes that one may believe pregnancy to be influenced by psychological factors even though this influence cannot be demonstrated. He finds no significant relationships between the psychological variables in question and the progress of the pregnancy, or between anxiety and pregnancy, but he does find such relationships between the variables themselves.

3. In order to avoid pre-selecting criteria (e.g. maturity or anxiety), which may often appear to be more or less arbitrarily chosen or defined, some workers have preferred to establish their scale once the case-histories are completed, basing it directly on their own data, and therefore upon material provided by the pregnant women themselves. This was attempted by Scott and Thompson (144) in their classification of the women as 'stable' and 'unstable'.

In the research carried out by the present writers (34 and the present work), the women were classified *a posteriori* according to the 'negative effects' exercised on their current situation by certain events and areas in their past life as a whole. The hypothesis, deliberately stated in the most general terms, was that in everyone's life there are handicaps, the sum total of which is influential, whatever types of reaction the woman may show. The scale adopted may appear a little oversimplified, but it has proved of practical value in enabling the data collected to be analysed. First, it was of use as a general measure of negativity; second, it demonstrated certain areas of negativity which occurred more frequently and exercised greater influence upon the course of the pregnancy and confinement; finally, it was by no means ineffective as a method of predicting the quality of confinements (cf. Chapter 5).

The procedure is open to criticism on the grounds of the (initially intentional) inclusiveness of the idea of negativity, which sums a whole range of different things; and also on account of the difficulty and possible inadequacy of the analysis of the methods of defence and adjustment employed by the women in relation to the burden of negativity to which their life has given rise. This counterbalancing factor is assessed through the nature of the woman's social, family, and professional adjustment, her contact with the research team, preparation for childbirth, and an overall clinical evaluation.

At this point, we come up against the serious difficulty that besets all classifications in this field, a difficulty that is particularly relevant to the prediction of confinements. Either the classification is one that enables comparisons to be made in quantitative terms, but is based upon superficial and more or less external or arbitrary factors which have little to do with what one knows and feels about pregnancy and confinement; or it is based upon a more general and deeper psychological point of view, in which case one has neither the conceptual nor the clinical material necessary to support and verify the hypotheses advanced. One is therefore more or less obliged to choose a middle path and run the double risk of oversimplifying and failing to come to grips with reality, and, in consequence, of not really being effective.

This conflict of levels of operation recurs constantly throughout the literature on pregnancy and confinement. Only certain forms of preparation for childbirth may perhaps claim to avoid it, and, even then, only to a certain extent and in certain ways; in fact, only in so far as preparation operates, at all stages of preparation and management of the confinement, at the level of learning or training, and is limited to a short period, appeals to conscious mechanisms, and keeps deep-lying problems at a distance, ignoring their existence. Even so, the problem cannot be completely avoided, as will presently appear when we consider recent works on preparation (Section IV, p. 275).

In every case, the dilemma is manifest in connexion with the prognosis of confinements. For it is indeed one of the aims of a physiological and psychological study of pregnant women, and their classification, to make possible some degree of predictability and understanding of confinements; and here different authors express very different opinions. The basic question is whether, if we know a woman's background and the history of her pregnancy, we can predict her confinement. Some say that it cannot be done, either because they have in fact no means of 'getting inside' confinements, or because their classification of the women is based on superficial observations of what is accessible to them in the course of their contacts with the women; with such methods of investigation it is difficult to predict the quality of confinements, although it is possible to deal effectively with fear and to

271

secure greater tolerance of the pain that is the inevitable accompaniment of childbirth. This is the conclusion arrived at by Matthews (103). In the case of other writers, their criteria, although they regard them as important, do not enable them to prognosticate about confinements (Brown, 22; Klein, Potter, and Dyk, 83; and Pavenstedt, 124).

With regard to Read's natural childbirth, some writers argue in a similar way, maintaining that preparation is very limited, that its effect is so superficial that there can be no guarantee as to what may happen, and that one simply does the best one can. This is the view of Scott and Thompson (144).

Others who practise preparation predict the probable course of the confinement on the basis of their knowledge of the women concerned: their state of fatigue, the conditions of their life, the history of their pregnancy, and in particular the quality of the preparation. It is as if there were two regions of unpredictability, the one biological, the other concerned with deep-lying psychological aspects such as profound regression, loss of control, etc. What in fact they are doing is predicting the firmness of the woman's self-control on the basis of learned behaviour. This position was often taken by practitioners of the PPM in the days when they attempted to use the rather oversimplified criteria defining nervous types for predicting confinements.

All these ambiguities and difficulties simply reflect the gulf between what childbirth expresses and stands for, and what we can discover about pregnancy with the methods at our disposal. Few authors deny that there is a relationship between personality and confinement, that confinement is both an ordeal imposed from without and a challenge to the individual personality, that it represents a particular form of self-expression on the part of the woman, though at a level and in ways difficult to define (Scott and Thompson, 144; Cappon, 25, etc.).

Starting from the position that confinement has genuinely expressive significance, Malcovati *et al.* (101) have reversed the question. Considering the two main and essentially different stages of childbirth (dilatation and expulsion), and the differences in behaviour that can always be seen during these stages, they trace the anxiety experienced and observed in the two stages to the two main types of primitive anxiety, according to psychoanalytic theory: depressive anxiety and aggressive anxiety. They use the expression, development, and operation of these two forms of anxiety experienced and manifested during childbirth to throw light retrospectively upon the problems of womanhood and pregnancy. This kind of work is well in line with the aims suggested elsewhere by Kammerer (cf. p. 267) – to collect fantasy material in order to throw light on underlying meanings. The idea of a revival of these two types of anxiety has not yet been conclusively demonstrated, but this line of research should be followed up, since it has the advantage of suggesting a means for the analysis of childbirth, giving it a special significance, and approaching it as an object for systematic investigation.

III. REJECTION AND ACCEPTANCE OF THE CHILD: MOTHER-CHILD RELATIONS

It was impossible in the present research to give adequate attention to the problem of the acceptance or rejection of the child by the pregnant woman, the parturient woman, or the young mother. This did, however, seem to be an important and puzzling phenomenon. Already present during childhood, such attitudes evolve rapidly during the different stages of pregnancy, and vary from one woman to another and from one pregnancy to another. They are accordingly as difficult to apprehend as to evaluate.

In the course of the present research, the writers were able to discern difficulties in acceptance of the child from the beginning of pregnancy by two methods: (a) the sociocultural approach, and (b) the symptomatological approach.

(a) *Sociocultural approach.* In a subsidiary research using the case-histories of the primiparae at the Hôpital Rothschild, the writers found a relationship between early and expressed rejection of a first baby (89 per cent of cases) and housing difficulties, showed how acute social problems and a deep-reaching psychological crisis interact, and traced out the symbolic ramifications of such interaction (36).

(b) *Approach in terms of symptoms.* It must be emphasized that we are here concerned with rejection expressed in words, and, of course, rejection of or desire for the child are even more important at the unconscious than at the conscious level. It is as if a variable period of adjustment to the presence of the baby is required, in which the woman becomes familiar with and imagines the child before actually experiencing it. The ambivalence of this period is revealed at the physical level by a crop of symptoms from the beginning of pregnancy, and frequently by disturbances of the body-image.

These disturbances have been examined from a psychoanalytic point of view by McConnell and Daston (99a), on the basis of interpretations of projective tests applied to a sample of pregnant women.

The baby becomes a living reality for the mother only when the *first movements* occur. A small-scale study which it is hoped to follow up (18) indicated that these first movements were instrumental in inducing the development of mother-child relations towards acceptance in 85 per cent of cases, towards greater ambivalence in 10 per cent of cases, and towards abnormal reactions of rejection in 5 per cent of cases. It may be said that if

273

nothing has happened before this critical moment, the relationship emerges in a very marked way when the baby is felt as a living entity but liable to death, dependent but moving, inside the mother's body but destined to emerge at birth, a part of her body and yet foreign to it, a promise and at the same time a threat.

In a fairly thorough study of the *vomiting of pregnancy*, the present writers demonstrated the predominant part played by certain kinds of ambivalence towards the child (32). Two samples of pregnant primiparae were compared, one consisting of those who vomited, the other of those who did not. The results indicated that the women who vomited were not those with the greatest practical difficulties, the most marked symptoms, or the greatest amount of illness; nor were they those who clearly accepted or rejected their child. The majority of the women who vomited had difficulty in accepting the child, and their pregnancy was characterized by alternation between strong desire for the child and equally strong rejection.

The most difficult problem in research of this kind is to establish criteria of acceptance and rejection for the different stages of pregnancy. But there is also another reason why this important concept has not received the full attention of the present writers, and has been the object only of exploratory research and preliminary reports, while the 'negativity grid' has been developed as a sensitive instrument for classifying women and predicting confinements. In the present state of our knowledge, the woman's attitude towards her child does not provide a basis for understanding and predicting the course of her confinement. This is because confinement may have very different meanings. A woman who wants and accepts her child may have a poor confinement because she resists being separated from him and expelling him into the outside world. On the other hand, a woman who rejects her child may have a short and easy labour because she wants to be separated from her child and to expel him as a bad object. Everything that the child represents for the mother, as a good or bad object, is thus involved here, alternatively or simultaneously, in a more or less conflict-laden way, varying with the different periods of pregnancy and the different stages of confinement. It is this emotional over-determination and these overtones of meaning that make it so difficult to grasp the realities of the situation simply in terms of acceptance or rejection of the child.

We are concerned here, however, with the inception of the early relations between mother and child, the establishment of which is a determining factor in their future life. The factors involved comprise not only, as already stated, the symptoms that may appear during the early months, vomiting, first movements, and verbal rejection from the beginning of pregnancy; but also the anxieties of the last weeks, the first look at the child, the first gestures, the first words, and the way in which these develop.

274

The first mother-child relations have been the object of some interesting studies, with regard to both the mother and the child. Pavenstedt (124), whose work has already been referred to, puts forward the view that the mother's immaturity is reflected in her child's behaviour. Mayer, Raimbault, and Raimbault (104), at the Hôpital Saint-Antoine, have attempted to trace in greater detail and in psychoanalytic terms the influence of maternal attitudes upon the child, and to establish a psychopathology for mother-child relations.

According to Helene Deutsch (44), a woman in labour always experiences two births – her own birth, which she relives, and that of the baby she is bringing into the world. For fifteen years or so, the study of this threefold relationship has received the attention of specialists in the psychology of women and in the problems of womanhood and motherhood.

Bibring (13) shows clearly the predominant influence of past and present relations between the young woman and her own mother on her reaction to pregnancy and on the development of her confinement, as well as on the establishment of mother-child relations.

Sylvia Markham (102), working along similar lines, shows by clinical case-studies that certain pathological deviations or difficulties in primiparae are related to mother-daughter fixation.

Finally, Racamier and his colleagues (133, 134), in an account of a new kind of psychiatric treatment, underline the importance of this threefold relationship throughout the study and treatment of the puerperal psychoses. In puerperal psychoses, the mother feels herself to be, and indeed is, dangerous to her child. This is so because she felt herself threatening and threatened in her relations with her own mother. Cure is achieved by providing her with concrete evidence that, with her baby in her arms, and the assistance of a psychotherapeutic team in the hospital setting, she does him no harm. These authors show that the establishment of 'maternalism' (the function of motherhood) has its origins in the mother's own experience as a girl. It is a complex function which is established gradually and is often vulnerable. Abnormality in respect of this function reflects an abnormal mother-daughter relationship. It is through the abnormal case that one can descry, as it were under magnification, the mechanism of a normal and fundamental relationship, which requires further detailed investigation.

IV. CURRENT PROBLEMS AND RECENT STUDIES OF PREPARATION FOR CHILDBIRTH

We shall limit ourselves here to mentioning recent work on painless childbirth and the controversies produced by the spread of preparation. There are already bibliographies and even critical reviews of all the literature published before 1958 (28), and the first chapter of this book, with its fifty references, also provides a fairly adequate documentation.

Mention may first of all be made of several practical textbooks which are more or less satisfactory in presentation and content. These are designed for pregnant women, with the twofold purpose of providing information and reassurance, as well as for staff engaged in giving preparation. There is, for example, a book by Goodrich (64), which purports to be both readable and attractive, and conveys in romanticized form a certain amount of useful information; but it spreads and perpetuates many confused ideas concerning the history of the P P M and natural childbirth, as also about the nature of pain, its role, and the attitudes to be encouraged confronting it. The French version of the book (65) certainly appears to be poorly adapted to the climate of thinking and the present position of the P P M in France.

On the other hand, the book by Bazelaire and Hersilie (8), based on twelve years' experience and practice of the P P M according to Dr Lamaze's methods, is a careful and up-to-date work, and contributes a helpful handbook for use in conjunction with preparation.

We must not omit to mention here two books by Vellay *et al.*, which have been in general use in preparation for childbirth for some years, both in France and elsewhere. Vellay was one of the earliest proponents of the P P M in France. Of these two books, one provides a concentrated account of all that needs to be known about painless childbirth (149); the other is a collection of documentary material – photographs and first-hand accounts by women who have had preparation. If the 'objectivity' of this work may still be questioned, the enthusiasm of the women and the subjective accounts they give of their experience are extremely convincing (150).

In the United States, Buxton (24), after spending a year in Europe, gives an account of his experiences concerning all the physical and psychological methods of preparation for childbirth. His aim is to inform the public, both medical and lay, on the various methods of preparation and their results. Buxton is especially aware of the fact that, in spite of the efforts of practitioners, no really objective assessment of results can be given because of the subjective nature of pain, and because it is impossible to carry out controlled experiments on one's subjects. He believes that women do in fact derive benefit from preparation, and thinks that this benefit should be generalized in the form of 'prenatal, natal, and neonatal hygiene'. This point of view, however, is debatable, since it pushes into the background the primary purpose of the method, psychological analgesia, for the sake of a degree of comfort for all women. It then becomes a question of either accepting the minimum goal of helping pregnant women, or insisting upon the maximum goal of making their confinements painless.

This is a major issue. All forms of preparation using methods that are spreading rapidly today vacillate between two extremes, and occupy an intermediate position. The alternative aims are, as has been indicated, to practise a form of very general mental hygiene which is already beneficial; or to offer the prospect of analgesia, a much more ambitious and difficult goal. The variety of designations (painless childbirth, psychoprophylactic method, natural childbirth, prepared childbirth, etc.) reflects differences in approach as well as the need felt by the various exponents to differentiate between their respective methods.

These problems, and many others, received particular attention at two congresses. The First International Congress of Psychosomatic Medicine and Childbirth, held in Paris in July 1962, was remarkable for the number of participants (over three hundred), and for the degree of awareness that it revealed, in twenty-two countries, of the problems of womanhood and motherhood. A number of papers read at this congress have been cited in this Appendix (Mead, Chertok, Malcovati, Raimbault, etc.). An issue of the *Revue de Médecine psychosomatique* (139) was devoted to it, and the complete *Proceedings* of this congress are also available (107).

Further, at the Congress of the Société française de Psychoprophylaxie obstétricale, held in Strasbourg in May 1963 (23), the majority of papers were concerned with the practice of the P P M. One series of papers dealt with mechanisms of uterine contraction and their relations with respiration (ventilation, oxygen therapy, respiratory rhythm, training in breathing) within the general framework of psychoprophylaxis. Another session comprised the more purely psychological papers. Several of these have already been referred to (Kammerer; Bonnaud and Revault d'Allonnes). To these should be added that of Mme Weill-Halle (155) on the role of family planning in preparation for motherhood; Mme Weill-Halle's presence at the congress is evidence of the common ground between birth control and planned parenthood, on the one hand, and preparation for childbirth, on the other.

This session inevitably led to a confrontation between psychoanalysts and practitioners of the method concerning the theoretical bases of the method, the level at which it operates, and the form that preparation should take. These discussions were in fact a continuation of those of an earlier period, referred to in Chapter 1, on psychotherapy and psychoprophylaxis, and illustrate the full import of the problems to which preparation for childbirth gives rise. A series of articles by Muldworf prepared the ground for, and followed up, these discussions. In 1962 he attempted to assess the psychological concepts underlying the P P M, by reference to Pavlovian theory and to psychology (112). More recently (113), he has attempted to trace the history of 'the myth of womanhood in psychoanalysis' and to dispose of it in a series of critical observations, which do not in fact settle the matter. The question remains open.

A trend towards the deepening and widening of psychological theories is reflected in a special number of the *Bulletin de la Société internationale de Psychoprophylaxie obstétricale*, which is devoted to the work of members of the Argentinian school. In an article by Koremblit and Chaves on 'The personal interview in psychoprophylaxis' (87), and in a paper by Bermudez on 'Fantasies and dreams of pregnant women' (12), the influence of psychoanalytic ideas is evident.

Complementary to the work of these two congresses, studies have been directed towards understanding the nature and development of preparation. Some of those engaged on the present research took up the questions of how information about the method was disseminated, of the motives of the women in respect of their acceptance or refusal of preparation, and especially of their reasons for *refusal*. At the present time, refusal is more unusual than acceptance, and indicates a psychological constellation, tentatively described in the relevant article, which includes social and philosophical aspects which are identified by means of an analysis of clinical material (34).

On the more strictly psychological aspects of preparation, an important article was published by Gressot in 1959 (66). According to Gressot, a confinement proceeds painlessly when 'all the obstetrical aspects are normal and, in addition, the effect of preparation is to make certain mental reactions to childbirth mutually compatible instead of antagonistic' (p. 43). The occurrence of suffering would, on this view, be linked with the presence of contradictory elements – conflicts within the personality or conflicts inherent in the social situation. Gressot has therefore studied the role of mental conflict towards the end of pregnancy and during confinement, fear with its basis in the unconscious and its social reinforcement, spontaneous defences against fear, different kinds of personality reaction to the stress of childbirth and their classification in terms of activity-passivity, dependence-independence, etc., the normal psychological significance of childbirth, and the psychological assistance provided by preparation both during preparation and during confinement, such as neutralization of conflicts, identification with the members of the group, transference to the person responsible for the preparation or to the staff, expression and neutralization of anxiety, and the influence of educational and interpersonal factors. This article demonstrates effectively how the study of psychological factors complements the understanding of the obstetrical and neurological aspects of preparation by emphasizing childbirth as a psychosomatic process, both a physical mechanism and an experience involving a considerable emotional outlay.

278

From a related, although somewhat different, point of view – that of drawing on psychoanalytic findings and attempting to define the place of prepared childbirth, to understand better its various implications – a special number of *Perspectives psychiatriques* (126) was devoted to 'The psychology and psychopathology of motherhood'. The issue as a whole surveyed the most important concepts of a dynamic psychology of femininity and motherhood. It contained, among other studies, those of Donnet, a paper on 'Pregnancy and confinement, their psychological organization' (48), and a study of the significance of preparation for childbirth entitled 'The myth of painless childbirth' (49). This consists of a critical analysis of preparation for childbirth as 'orthodoxy', i.e. as conforming to the image it presents, and then as a 'Trojan horse', i.e. as calling on an ethic and norms that it does not make explicit. These two aspects – the explicit and the implicit – of preparation for childbirth are compared with psychoanalytic findings and what is established is their agreement, in general and on a majority of points – an agreement that, with the current trend of ideas, should become still more apparent in the future.

Finally, in 1966 Chertok published a paper (English version (33a)) in which he considered the position of preparation, dealing with both its spread and the theoretical problems and research to which it gives rise.

Preparation has spread to some extent almost all over the world, but particularly in France and the Latin countries, whereas it has encountered considerable resistance in the United States. The traditional pattern of American obstetrics has been against the spread of preparation, as Buxton's work, already referred to (24), indicates. Since both women and doctors are used to putting their faith in drugs and anaesthesia, the problem of pain receives little attention, and there does not appear to be any need for a special method of suppressing it. No doubt, also, the American practitioners have been opposed to prepared childbirth as a result of the unconscious resistance that is always encountered among doctors when psychological factors are introduced into treatment in their own special field. This opposition is strengthened by the fact that in the United States the presence of a doctor is the rule for all confinements, and the doctors would not have enough time to devote to each patient if they had to apply the methods of prepared childbirth (it should be remembered that there are no midwives in the United States). This explains why, in spite of the possible harmful effects of systematic anaesthesia (at least as far as the foetus is concerned), and in spite of the desire expressed by some women to experience the birth as fully as possible, systematic methods of preparation are not felt to be necessary either by the women or by the doctors. Thus, although Helene Deutsch (44) favours preparation, the American psychoanalyst Heiman (68a) rejects prepared childbirth on the grounds that it deprives the woman of beneficial regressive

279

episodes, and may stimulate pathological aspects of her personality; according to him, in the United States, women who want preparation are most frequently psychologically disturbed and would run the risk of being even more so afterwards.

Recent information, however, indicates that the instruction of pregnant women is beginning to spread. In some centres, preparation is given by Read's method; in others, psychoprophylaxis is used. The word 'psychoprophylaxis' is becoming progressively more common in the United States. This method is sought particularly in the Northern states by women belonging to groups that have recently moved from Europe. It is practised, under private supervision, by women from the highest social classes who are able to go against established opinion. These women also appear to accept their womanhood better, and in particular to be more ready to breast-feed.

On the whole, the number of expectant mothers who use preparation is extremely small in the United States. This is a somewhat paradoxical situation, since the method reflects the psychosomatic point of view, which is well developed in that country.

In France, the position of prepared childbirth is particularly favourable, and it is estimated that roughly 50 per cent of women take advantage of it. This success is due to a surprising conjunction of influence from both the political Left and the Catholic church. The PPM, introduced into France by Lamaze on his return from the USSR in 1952, was, to begin with, practised by a minority of women politically involved in Leftist organizations. They were activated by powerful ideological motives. By choosing prepared childbirth, they felt that they were executing a pioneering act which should help to promote the ideas in which they believed – the futility of suffering, confidence in science and its techniques, the demystification of sex, the liberation of women, and the value of awareness and activity.

The Catholic church, for its part, was soon won over to the PPM. Several French cardinals were the first to pronounce in its favour. Official approval was given in January 1956 by the Pope's announcement of his position in his address to the International Congress of Gynaecology and Obstetrics. In this well-documented statement, the Pope explained the Pavlovian principles underlying the PPM and unreservedly supported the practice of the method, although it derived from a country with a materialist ideology. Thus Catholic women, and especially those in Latin countries, were confirmed in their decision to have preparation for childbirth, in the name of personalistic Christian morality emphasizing the humanization of natural functions, respect for maternity and woman's nature, the dignity of effort, and the value of self-mastery.

Yet another factor would appear to have favoured the spread of preparation in France and in Europe in general: the obstetrical tradition has been in favour of only moderate use of anaesthetics and, used to the idea that suffering was associated with the process of giving birth, women seized the opportunity offered them of a safe method of analgesia.

On the theoretical level, Chertok's paper indicates the difficulties facing the different methods if they are to explain scientifically the mechanisms of psychological analgesia. The author outlines the various controversies and affirms that opposition between activity and passivity is today the main point at issue in theoretical discussions. Nicolaiev and his collaborators (120), and with them the whole French school, reproach Read's method with relying on passivity in various forms. Nicolaiev declares that 'isolation from the outside world, a raising of the threshold of awareness and feelings of ecstasy may make analgesia possible, but at the cost of what is a genuinely pathological state of the higher nervous system, whereas the PPM, by promoting activity, contributes to the strengthening of the higher nervous system'. Nicolaiev rejects any form of passivity, whether effected by psychotropic drugs which reduce vigilance, by relaxation which involves a raising of the threshold of awareness, or finally by panting. On the other hand, he recommends everything that can raise the threshold of awareness and reinforce higher nervous activity – information, rhythmic breathing, physical exercises, and so on.

This uncompromising rejection of any kind of passivity in the use of a method derived from the hypno-suggestive method may seem curious. For the PPM, passivity appears as undesirable and almost sinful. This may be because a passive attitude on the part of the expectant mother obliges the physician to take charge of her and thereby assume additional responsibility. Feminine passivity may also have a certain erotic connotation. In this case, the condemnation of passivity would represent a rationalization of the resistances experienced by the physician to interpersonal involvement, of which the hypnotic relationship is the most highly developed form. Such resistances have marked the history of psychotherapy for two centuries.

It would therefore appear: (i) that the maintaining of an opposition between activity and passivity, between activation and inhibition, between the passive aspects of Read's method and the active aspects of the PPM, has no more than verbal significance and has no constructive contribution to offer; and (ii) that to use an exclusively physiological vocabulary to describe psychological phenomena (lacking an adequate experimental basis) contributes nothing to the understanding of the problem. A viable theory of drugless analgesia can be established only on the basis of empirical research directed at the mechanisms of attention and hypnotic analgesia, at both the neurological and the psychological level.

Since this paper by Chertok, there has appeared an article by Lebedev (95a) which makes one wonder whether the PPM may not be undergoing an evolution in its orientation. Before examining this article, it will be useful to outline, with the help of a detailed article by Chertok (33), the main stages in the evolution of the PPM in the Soviet Union. These are characterized by a remarkable parallelism in both terminology and techniques of preparation.

When he propounded the method in 1949, the psychiatrist Velvovski referred to it by the name of *psychotherapeutic method of obstetrical analgesia*. In 1950 the obstetrician Nicolaiev proposed the term *psychoprophylaxis*, which was accepted. In the same year, there took place the famous joint meeting of the Academies of Sciences and of Medicine of the Soviet Union, which laid down the principle that psychology was dependent upon physiology, that there was no independent discipline of psychology, and that psychology was subordinate to physiology. In 1951 the method, recognized by the Ministry of Health, was officially established, and it was this method that was introduced and widely disseminated in France by Lamaze.

At this time, psychoprophylaxis was regarded as a 'mental' method and was opposed to Read's method, considered as a 'physical' method, i.e. consisting mainly of physical exercises. The practice of physical exercises, rejected in both France and the Soviet Union, was the subject of a number of controversies at the time (cf. Chapter 1).

In 1956 psychology started to acquire independence of physiology (an independence that was to be confirmed, in 1962, by the Moscow Congress on Philosophical Problems of Higher Nervous Activity and Psychology). In 1959 Nicolaiev (117) introduced gymnastics into preparation. In 1961 (119) he insisted on its importance and also introduced other physical agents – ultra-violet rays, hydrotherapy, and so on. These physical agents were supposed to increase bodily resistance and cortical tonus, and to reinforce the suggestive element in the method. Nicolaiev then suggested that the PPM be called *psychophysioprophylaxis*.

In 1961 Rechetova (138a) published a new programme of preparation comprising three aspects: dietetics, the physical agents already recommended by Nicolaiev, and classical psychoprophylaxis.

In 1966 there appeared the article by Lebedev (95a), professor of obstetrics at Moscow, reporting the results of an investigation of 4,000 cases and recommending certain modifications in preparation. He called his method *physiopsychoprophylaxis*, thus giving pride of place to the prefix *physio* and the physical agents, in accordance with the spirit and content of his method. Preparation as practised by him depends upon the observation that, if physical elements are added, the effectiveness of the method is increased. Consequently, preparation, which extends over the whole of pregnancy, confinement, and the post-partum period, includes many sessions of medical gymnastics, exposure to ultra-violet rays, 'sanitary hygiene', etc. Gymnastics are presented as not only beneficial for the mother but also excellent for the foetus, affecting and accelerating foetal circulation. Ultra-violet rays are said to have a bactericidal action, confirmed by experiments on animals, etc. Psychoprophylaxis properly speaking only really appears during the third period of pregnancy (32nd to 40th week) and is reduced to four sessions. The total proportion is therefore four sessions of psychoprophylaxis against about fifty sessions of ultra-violet rays and an even larger number of sessions of physical exercises.

The author reports excellent results with his method, and compares these with results for unprepared women, but he makes no comparisons with a control group consisting of women prepared by the classical PPM. The present writers are not aware whether this method, in which psychoprophylaxis is submerged by a profusion of physical agents, is spreading in the USSR, but are inclined to doubt it, in spite of the prestige that Lebedev himself probably enjoys.

There is, however, an interesting theoretical, practical, and terminological development of the method in the USSR. The crucial point is the prefix *psycho*, which is displaced at will, while its importance decreases simultaneously. The reason is that it expresses the personal, relational element which, in the Soviet Union as elsewhere, arouses resistances in the medical world.

To sum up, at the present time the United States, the leading country in psychosomatic medicine, stands aloof from psychoprophylaxis, for cultural, medical, and psychological reasons. In the Soviet Union, where the method was first introduced, it is spreading, but it is undergoing modifications that are tending to deprive it of its properly psychological aspects. Is it not reasonable to suppose that, in both cases, there is resistance to the aspect of psychological involvement, i.e. to the relational and personal factors involved in the method?

It would appear that, in France, those concerned are on the way to finding a reasonable balance, taking into consideration the psychological elements which are so important in preparation. This is probably due to the specific historical and cultural conditions which Chertok has described in his paper (33a).

Bibliography

1. ABRAHAM, K. (1922). Manifestations of the female castration complex. *Int. J. Psycho-Anal.*, **3**, 1–29.

2. ABRAMSON, M., and HERON, W. T. (1950). Objective evaluation of hypnosis in obstetrics: preliminary report. *Amer. J. Obstet. Gynec.*, **59**, 1069–1074.

3. AJURIAGUERRA, J. DE (1959). L'intégration de la douleur. Pp. 1–15 in Aboulker, Chertok, and Sapir (eds.), *Analgésie psychologique en obstétrique.* Paris: Pergamon Press.

4. ANGELERGUES, R. (1954). La conception pavlovienne de la douleur dans l'accouchement. *Rev. nouv. Méd.*, **1**, 3, 9–32.

5. ANGELERGUES, R. (1960). Évolution de la méthode psychoprophylactique. Ire partie. *Bull. Soc. franç. Psychoprophyl. obstét.*, **2**, 115–131.

6. ASTAKHOV, S. N., and BESKROVNAIA, N. I. (1952). Nach opyt obezbolivania v rodakh metodom slovesnovo vozdieistvia na beremiennouiov i rojdenitsou (Painless childbirth by the verbal activity method in pregnant and parturient women). Pp. 48–54 in (38) (in Russian).

7. BALINT, M. (1957). *The Doctor, his Patient and the Illness.* London: Pitman Medical; New York: International Universities Press.

8. BAZELAIRE, S., and HERSILIE, R. (1963). *Maternité (fécondation, grossesse, accouchement).* Paris: La Table ronde.

9. BELOCHAPKO, P. A., and FOI, A. M. (1954). *Obezbolivanie i Ousskorenie Rodov (Analgesia and the Acceleration of Labour).* Moscow: Medguiz (in Russian).

10. BENEDEK, T. (1952). *Psychosexual Functions in Women.* New York: Ronald Press.

11. BENEDEK, T. (1960). The organisation of the reproduction drive. *Int. J. Psycho-Anal.*, **41**, 1–15.

12. BERMUDEZ, J. R. (1964). Imagination et rêves dans des groupes de femmes enceintes. *Bull. Soc. int. Psychoprophyl. obstét.*, **6**, 109–125.

13. BIBRING, G. L. (1959). Some considerations on the psychological processes in pregnancy. *Psychoanal. Study Child*, **14**, 113–121.

14. BIBRING, G. L., THOMAS, F., and DWYER, M. (1961). Study of the psychological processes in pregnancy and of the earliest mother-child relationship. I: Some propositions and comments. *Psychoanal. Study Child*, **16**, 9–24.

15. BIBRING, G. L., THOMAS, F., and DWYER, M. (1961). Study of the psychological processes in pregnancy and of the earliest mother-child relationship. II: Methodological considerations. *Psychoanal. Study Child*, **16**, 25–72.

16. BONAPARTE, M. (1935). Passivité, masochisme et féminité. Pp. 26–34 in *Psychanalyse et Biologie*. Paris: Presses Universitaires de France, 1952.

17. BONAPARTE, M. (1957). *De la sexualité de la femme*. Paris: Presses Universitaires de France.

18. BONNAUD, M., and REVAULT D'ALLONNES, C. (1963). Vécu psychologique des premiers mouvements de l'enfant. *Bull. Soc. franç. Psychoprophyl. obstét.*, **15**, 43–47.

19. BRENMAN, M. (1951). Perception of pain and some factors that modify it. Pp. 103–122 in H. Abramson (ed.), *Problems of Consciousness*. New York: Josiah Macy Foundation.

20. BRISSET, C. (1963). Le culturalisme en psychiatrie (étude critique). *Evol. psychiat.*, **18**, 369–405.

21. BRISSET, C., and HELD, J. P. (1955). Accidents psychiatriques de la grossesse et de la puerpéralité. *Encycl. méd.-chir.*, art. 37660 A 10, Psychiatrie, **2**, 1–8.

22. BROWN, L. B. (1964). Anxiety in pregnancy. *Brit. J. med. Psychol.*, **37**, 47–58.

23. *Bulletin de la Société française de Psychoprophylaxie obstétricale* (1963). Actes du 5ᵉ Congrès. **14** (June) and **15** (September).

24. BUXTON, L. (1962). *A Study of Psychophysical Methods for Relief of Childbirth Pain*. Philadelphia and London: Saunders.

25. CAPPON, D. (1954). Some psychodynamic aspects of pregnancy. *Canad. med. Ass. J.*, **70**, 147–156.

26. CHAPMAN, C. (1957). Psychosomatic factors in obstetrics and gynaecology. *Med. J. Aust.*, **1**, 379–380.

26a. CHASSEGUET-SMIRGEL, J. (1964). *Recherches psychanalytiques sur la sexualité féminine* (with C. J. Luquet-Parat, B. Grunberger, J. McDougall, M. Torok, and C. David). Paris: Payot.

27. CHERTOK, L. (1956). Étude de la psycho-prophylaxie des douleurs de l'accouchment. *Sem. Hôp. Paris*, **32**, 2619–2626.

28. CHERTOK, L. (1959). *Psychosomatic Methods in Painless Childbirth*. London: Pergamon Press.

29. CHERTOK, L. (1959). Sur les rapports entre l'accouchement naturel et l'accouchement psychoprophylactique. *Praxis*, **44**, 1002–1004.

30. CHERTOK, L. (1961). Relaxation and psychosomatic methods of preparation for childbirth. *Amer. J. Obstet. Gynec.*, **82**, 262–267.

31. CHERTOK, L. (1963). Theories of psychoprophylaxis in obstetrics (prophylaxis or therapy). *Amer. J. Psychiat.*, **119**, 1152–1159.

32. CHERTOK, L. (1963). Vomiting and the wish to have a child. *Psychosom. Med.*, **25**, 13–18.

33. CHERTOK, L. (1966). Déclin de l'accouchement sans douleur? *Concours méd.*, **26**, 4621–4628.

33a. CHERTOK, L. (1967) Psychosomatic methods of preparation for childbirth: spread of the methods, theory and research. *Amer. J. Obstet. Gynec.*, **98**, 698–707.

34. CHERTOK, L., DONNET, J. L., REVAULT D'ALLONNES, C., and BONNAUD, M. (1961). Sur les motivations du refus de l'ASD. *Bull. Soc. int. Psychoprophyl. obstét.*, **3**, 1–19.

35. CHERTOK, L., DONNET, J. L., BONNAUD, M., and BORELLI-VINCENT, M. (1962). Éléments psychologiques du pronostic de l'accouchement. Pp. 337–341 in (107).

36. CHERTOK, L., and REVAULT D'ALLONNES, C. (1964). Habitation et grossesse. *Hyg. ment.*, **53**, 109–126.

37. Congress in Kiev on the advancement of psychoprophylactic preparation for labour, 10–14 February 1956. Papers published in *Akush. i Ginek.*, Moscow, May–June 1956, **3**, 3–84 (in Russian).

38. Congress in Leningrad on obstetrical analgesia, 29–31 January 1951. Proceedings published in *Obezbolivanie y Rodakh* (*Obstetrical Analgesia*). Moscow: Akad. Med. Nauk, SSSR, 1952 (in Russian). Translated into German as *Schmerzausschaltung bei der Geburt*. Berlin: VEB-Verlag, 1953.

39. DAVIDENKOV, S. N. (1952). Comment at Leningrad Congress. P. 71 in (38) (in Russian).

40. DAVIDS, A., and DE VAULT, S. (1960). Use of the TAT and human figure drawings in research on personality, pregnancy and perception. *J. project. Tech.*, **24**, 362–365.

41. DAVIDS, A., DE VAULT, S., and TALMADGE, M. (1961). Anxiety, pregnancy and childbirth abnormalities. *J. consult. Psychol.*, **28**, 74–77.

42. DAVIDS, A., DE VAULT, S., and TALMADGE, M. (1961). Psychological study of emotional factors in pregnancy: a preliminary report. *Psychosom. Med.*, **23**, 93–103.

43. DEUTSCH, H. (1930). The significance of masochism in the mental life of women. Pp. 195–207 in R. Fliess (ed.), *A Psychoanalytic Reader*. New York: International Universities Press, 1949; London: Hogarth Press, 1950.

44. DEUTSCH, H. (1944). *The Psychology of Women: A Psychoanalytic Interpretation*. 2 vols. London: Heinemann; New York: Grune & Stratton.

45. DEUTSCH, H., and FREUD, S. (1925). The psychology of women in relation to the function of reproduction. Pp. 165–179 in R. Fliess (ed.), *A Psychoanalytic Reader*. New York: International Universities Press, 1949; London: Hogarth Press, 1950.

46. DOLINE, A. O., and SALGANNIK, G. M. (1956). Fiziologicheskiie ossnovi psikhoprofilakticheskoi podgotovki (The physiological bases of psychoprophylactic preparation for labour). Pp. 47–62 in (37) (in Russian).

47. DONIGEVICH, M. I. (1955). *Metod Psikhoprofilaktiki Boliei v Rodakh (The Psychoprophylactic Method of Painless Childbirth)*. Kiev: Gosmedizdat (in Russian).

48. DONNET, J. L. (1963). La grossesse et l'accouchement, leur régime psychologique. *Perspect. Psychiat.*, **4**, 11–16.

49. DONNET, J. L. (1963). Le mythe de l'ASD. *Perspect. Psychiat.*, **4**, 43–49.

50. DONOVAN, P., and LANDISBERG, S. (1953). Some psychological observations of 'Educated Childbirth'. *N.Y. State J. Med.*, **6**, 2504–2510.

51. DUFRENNE, M. (1953). *La notion de personnalité de base et son contexte dans l'anthropologie américaine*. Paris: Presses Universitaires de France.

52. ERIKSON, E. H. (1950). *Childhood and Society*. New York: Norton. Rev. edn., New York: Norton, 1963; London: Hogarth Press, 1965.

53. FERENCZI, S. (1924). *Thalassa: A Theory of Genitality*. New York: Psychoanalytic Quarterly, 1934.

54. FERREIRA, A. J. (1960). The pregnant woman's emotional attitude and its reflection on the newborn. *Amer. J. Orthopsychiat.*, **30**, 553.

55. FERREIRA GOMEZ, A. (1955). Los metodos psicofisicos en la analgesia del parto normal (Psychophysical methods in analgesia in normal childbirth). *Rev. esp. obstet. Ginec.*, **14**, 289–301 (in Spanish).

56. FOX, H. (1958). Narcissistic defences during pregnancy. *Psychoanal. Quart.*, **27**, 340–358.

57. FREUD, S. (1914). On narcissism: an introduction. Standard Edition, Vol. XIV. London: Hogarth Press.

58. FREUD, S. (1923). *The Ego and the Id*. Standard Edition, Vol. XIX. London: Hogarth Press.

59. FREUD, S. (1927). Some psychological consequences of the anatomical difference between the sexes. *Int. J. Psycho-Anal.*, **8**, 133–142.

60. FREUD, S. (1932). Concerning the sexuality of women. *Psychoanal. Quart.*, **1**, 191–209.

61. FREUD, S. (1933). The psychology of women. In *New Introductory Lectures on Psycho-analysis*. Standard Edition, Vol. XXII. London: Hogarth Press.
62. FREUD, S. *Complete Psychological Works*. Standard Edition. 24 vols. London: Hogarth Press, 1953–1966.
63. FRIES, M. (1941). Mental hygiene in pregnancy, delivery and puerperium. *Ment. Hyg.*, **25**, 221–236.
64. GOODRICH, F. W. (1950). *Natural Childbirth. A Manual for Expectant Parents*. New York: Prentice-Hall.
65. GOODRICH, F. W. (1954). *Comment accoucher sans douleur*. French version by Dr Chevalier. Paris: Marabout-Service.
66. GRESSOT, M. (1959). Aspects psychologiques de l'ASD. *Bull. Soc. int. Psychoprophyl. obstét.*, **1**, 43–75.
67. HARRIES, J., and HUGHES, T. (1958). Enumeration of the cravings of some pregnant women. *Brit. med. J.* (2), 39–40.
68. HEARDMAN, H. (1951). *Physiotherapy in Obstetrics and Gynaecology (including Education for Childbirth)*. Edinburgh: E. & S. Livingstone.
68a. HEIMAN, M. B. (1965). A psychoanalytic view of pregnancy. Pp. 473–511 in Rowinsky and Guttmacher (eds.), *Medical, Surgical and Gynecologic Complications of Pregnancy*. Baltimore: Williams & Wilkins.
69. HERNANDEZ-PEON, R., SCHERRER, H., and JOUVET, M. (1956). Modification of electric activity in cochlear nucleus during 'attention' in unanesthetized cats. *Science*, **123**, 331–332.
70. HERNON QUIJADA. Une grossesse et un accouchement suivis psychanalytiquement. Rapports réflexo-analytiques. Considérations psychosomatiques sur le foetus. (Unpublished, personal communication.)
71. HOOKE, J., and MARKS, P. L. (1962). MMPI characteristic of pregnancy. *J. clin. Psychol.*, **18**, 316–317.
72. HORNEY, K. (1924). On the genesis of castration complex of women. *Int. J. Psycho-Anal.*, **5**, 50–65.
73. HORNEY, K. (1933). Psychogenic factors in functional female disorders. *Amer. J. Obstet. Gynec.*, **25**, 694–704.
74. JACOBSON, E. (1938). *Progressive Relaxation*. Chicago: University of Chicago Press.
75. JACOBSON, E. (1954). Relaxation methods in labor: a critique of current techniques in natural childbirth. *Amer. J. Obstet. Gynec.*, **67**, 1035–1048.
76. JONES, E. (1927). The early development of female sexuality. Pp. 556–570 in *Papers on Psycho-analysis*. London: Baillière, Tindall & Cox, 1950.

77. JONES, E. (1935). Early female sexuality. Pp. 605–616 in *Papers on Psycho-analysis*. London: Baillière, Tindall & Cox, 1950.

78. JONES, E. (1942). Psychology and childbirth. *Lancet* (1), 695–696.

79. JORDANIA, I. F. (1952). Piat liet psikhoprofilakticheskoi podgotovki beremiennikh k rodam (Experience of the psychoprophylactic régime in a maternity unit). *Akush. i Ginek.*, 4 (in Russian). (French translation in *Cah. Méd. Sov.*, 1953, 1, 171–180.)

80. JOUVET, M. (1957). Étude neurophysiologique chez l'homme de quelques mécanismes sous-corticaux de l'attention. *Psychologie française*, 2, 254–260.

81. KAMMERER, T. (1963). La psychologie de la douleur. *Bull. Soc. franç. Psychoprophyl. obstét.*, 15, 115–122.

82. KLEIN, M. (1932). *The Psycho-analysis of Children*. London: Hogarth Press.

83. KLEIN, H., POTTER, H., and DYK, R. (1950). *Anxiety in pregnancy and childbirth*. (Psychosom. Med. Monograph.) New York: Hoeber.

84. KOGERER, H. (1922). Die posthypnotische Geburtsanalgesie (Post-hypnotic analgesia in childbirth). *Wiener klin. Wschr.*, 23, 513–517; 24, 538–540; 25, 558–561 (in German).

85. KONSTANTINOV, V. I. (1956). Teoria i praktika psikhoprofilakticheskoi podgotovki k rodam beremiennikh (Theory and practice of psychoprophylactic preparation for childbirth). Pp. 11–17 in (37) (in Russian).

86. KOPIL-LEVINA, Z. A. (1940). Metodika obezbolivania rodov slovesnim vnoucheniem (The verbal suggestion method of obstetrical analgesia). Pp. 34–65 in K. I. Platonov (ed.), *Voprossi Psikhoterapii v Akoucherstvie* (*Problems of Psychotherapy in Obstetrics*). Kharkov (in Russian).

87. KOREMBLIT, E., and CHAVES, T. M. DE (1961). L'entrevue personnelle en psychoprophylaxie. *Bull. Soc. int. Psychoprophyl. obstét.*, 6, 69–83.

88. KROGER, W. S. (1953). 'Natural childbirth': is Read's method of 'natural childbirth' waking hypnotism? *Brit. J. med. Hypnot.*, 1–15.

89. KROGER, W. S., and DE LEE, T. (1943). The use of hypnoidal state as an amnestic, analgesic and anesthetic agent in obstetrics. *Amer. J. Obstet. Gynec.*, 46, 655–661.

90. LAMAZE, F. (1956). *Qu'est-ce que l'accouchement sans douleur par la méthode psychoprophylactique? Ses principes, sa réalisation, ses résultats.* Paris: Savoir et Connaître.

91. LAMPL-DE GROOT, J. (1927). The evolution of the oedipus complex in women. Pp. 180–194 in R. Fliess (ed.), *A Psychoanalytic Reader*.

289

New York: International Universities Press, 1949; London: Hogarth Press, 1950.

92. LAMPL-DE GROOT, J. (1933). Problems of femininity. *Psychoanal. Quart.*, **2**, 489–518.

93. LANGER, M. (1944). Algunas aportaciones a la psicologia de la menstruación (Some observations on the psychology of menstruation). *Rev. Psicoanal.*, Buenos Aires, **5**, 93–99 (in Spanish).

94. LANGER, M. (1951). *Maternidad y Sexo* (*Motherhood and Sex*). Buenos Aires: Nova Biblioteca Psicoanal. (in Spanish).

95. LAWTON, J., and SISKO, F. (1961). Mental health aspects of pregnancy. *Psychiat. Quart. Suppl.*, **35**, 304–311.

95a. LEBEDEV, A. A. (1966). Fisiopsikhoprofilaktika v akoucherstvie (Physiopsychoprophylaxis in obstetrics). *Akush. i Ginek.*, **1**, 39–44 (in Russian).

96. LE SENNE, R. (1963). *Traité de caractérologie.* Paris: Presses Universitaires de France.

97. LEVIT, I. B., and RABINOVICH, F. I. (1955). Psikhoprofilakticheskii metod obezbolivania rodov (Psychoprophylaxis of the pains of childbirth). *Akush. i Ginek.*, **1**, 33–36 (in Russian).

98. LIÉBEAULT, A. A. (1887). Emploi de la suggestion hypnotique en obstétrique. *Rev. Hypnot.*, May, 328–332.

99. MACCAMMON, C. H. (1951). A study of 475 pregnancies in American Indian women. *Amer. J. Obstet. Gynec.*, **61**, 1159–1168.

99a. MCCONNELL, O. L., and DASTON, P. (1961). Body images changes in pregnancy. *J. project. Tech.*, **25**, 451–456.

100. MACK BRUNSWICK, R. (1940). The pre-oedipal phase of the libido development. Pp. 231–253 in R. Fliess (ed.), *A Psychoanalytic Reader.* New York: International Universities Press, 1949; London: Hogarth Press, 1950.

101. MALCOVATI, P., FORNARI, F., and MIRAGLIA, F. (1962). Les angoisses primaires chez la femme lors de l'accouchement. Pp. 381–386 in (107).

102. MARKHAM, S. (1961). A comparative evaluation of psychotic and non-psychotic reaction to childbirth. *Amer. J. Orthopsychiat.*, **31**, 565–578.

103. MATTHEWS, A. E. B. (1961). Behaviour patterns in labour: a study of consecutive patients. *J. Obstet. Gynaec. Brit. Comm.*, **68**, 862–874.

104. MAYER, M., RAIMBAULT, E., and RAIMBAULT, G. (1962). Maternité pathologique et troubles psychosomatiques de l'enfant. Pp. 393–397 in (107).

105. MEAD, M. (1935). *Sex and Temperament in Three Primitive Societies.* London: Routledge.

106. MEAD, M., and NEWTON, N. (1962). Conception, pregnancy, labour and the puerperium in cultural perspective. Pp. 51–54 in (107).

107. *Médecine psychosomatique et Maternité* (Proceedings of the First International Congress of Psychosomatic Medicine and Childbirth, Paris, 8–12 July 1962). Paris: Gauthier-Villars, 1965.

108. MENNINGER, W. C. (1943). The emotional factors in pregnancy. *Bull. Menninger Clin.*, 7, 15–24.

109. MULDWORF, B. (1959). Les bases théoriques de l'accouchement sans douleur par la méthode psychoprophylactique. *Bull. Soc. franç. Psychoprophyl. obstét.*, 1, 8–32.

110. MULDWORF, B. (1960). Pédagogie et psychothérapie dans la méthode psychoprophylactique d'accouchement sans douleur. *Bull. Soc. franç. Psychoprophyl. obstét.*, June, special issue, 3–10.

111. MULDWORF, B. (1961). Bilan théorique et évolution des idées en psychoprophylaxie. *Bull. Soc. franç. Psychoprophyl. obstét.*, 6, 59–73.

112. MULDWORF, B. (1962). Mentalité et psychologie chez la femme enceinte. *Bull. Soc. franç. Psychoprophyl. obstét.*, 10, 45–64.

113. MULDWORF, B. (1964). Féminité et psychologie féminine selon la psychanalyse. *Bull. Soc. franç. Psychoprophyl. obstét.*, 18, 3–18.

114. NEWTON, N. (1955). *Maternal Emotions: a Study of Women's Feelings toward Menstruation, Pregnancy, Childbirth, Breast Feeding, Infant Care and Other Aspects of their Femininity.* New York: Hoeber.

115. NEWTON, N. (1963). Emotions of pregnancy. *Clin. Obstet. Gynec.*, 6, 639–668.

116. NEWTON, N. (1964). Some aspects of primitive childbirth. *J. Amer. med. Assoc.*, 188, 261–264.

117. NICOLAIEV, A. P. (1953). *Ocherki Teorii i Praktiki Obezbolivania Rodov (Theory and Practice of Obstetrical Analgesia)*. 2nd edn. 1959. Moscow: Medguiz (in Russian).

118. NICOLAIEV, A. P. (1957). Osnovnie itogi tvorcheskovo primenienia fiziologicheskovo ouchenia I. P. Pavlov v akoucherstvie i gine-kologii (Basic problems in the application of the physiological teachings of Pavlov in obstetrics and gynaecology). *Akush. i Ginek.*, 5, 42–57 (in Russian).

119. NICOLAIEV, A. P. (1961). Sostojanie i perspektivy obezbolivania rodov v SSSR (The present state and prospects for obstetrical analgesia in the USSR). *Vestnik Ak. med. nauk SSSR*, 2, 64–69 (in Russian).

120. NICOLAIEV, A. P. (ed.) (1964). *Obezbolivanie Rodov (Obstetrical Analgesia)*. Leningrad: Meditzina (in Russian).

121. OETTINGEN, VON (1921). Zur Frage der schmerzlosen Geburt (On painless childbirth). *Muenchener med. Wschr.*, **51**, 1654–1655 (in German).

122. PARKS, J. (1951). Emotional reactions to pregnancy. *Amer. J. Obstet. Gynec.*, **62**, 339–345.

123. PAVENSTEDT, E. (1959). *Progress Report.* USPHS grant application, March 1959. (Unpublished.)

124. PAVENSTEDT, E. (1964). *The effect of maternal maturity and immaturity on child development.* USPHS grant application, September 1959 – August 1964. (Unpublished.)

125. PAVLOV, I. P. (1951). *Polnoie Sobranie Sochinenii* (Complete Works). Academy of Sciences of the USSR. 6 vols. (in Russian).

126. *Perspectives psychiatriques* (1963). Psychologie et psychopathologie de la maternité. Paris, September, **4**.

127. PETROV-MASLAKOV, M. A., and ZACHEPITZKI, R. A. (1953). *Psikhoprofilaktika Rodovikh Boliei* (*Psychoprophylaxis of the Pains of Childbirth*). Moscow: Medguiz (in Russian).

128. PLATONOV, K. I. (1937). Psikhicheskiie faktori pri obezbolivanii rodov (Psychological factors in obstetrical analgesia). *Akush. i Ginek.*, **9–10**, 93–99 (in Russian).

129. PLESHETTE, N., CHASE, J., and ASCH, S. S. (1956). A study of anxieties during pregnancy, labor, the early and late puerperium. *Bull. N.Y. Acad. Med.*, **32**, 436–455.

130. PLOTITCHER, V. A. (1954). Lectures 9, 10, 11, and 12. Pp. 168–226 in (152) (in Russian).

131. PRILL, H. J. (1956). Methoden psychischer Geburtsschmerzerleichterung (Psychological methods of lessening the pains of childbirth). *Z. Geburtsh. Gynaek.*, 211–229 (in German).

132. RACAMIER, P. C. (1955). Maladies des fonctions reproductrices de la femme. *Encycl. méd.-chir.*, art. 37490 C 10, Psychiatrie, **2**, 1–8.

133. RACAMIER, P. C. (1959). Les nourrissons avec leur mère à l'Hôpital psychiatrique. *Vie sociale et traitement*, **25**, 1–5.

134. RACAMIER, P. C., SENS, C., and CARRETIER, L. (1961). La mère et l'enfant dans les psychoses du post-partum. *Évol. psychiat.*, **4**, 525–570.

135. RANK, O. (1929). *The Trauma of Birth.* London: Kegan Paul.

136. RAPAPORT, D. (1951). Perception of pain and some factors that modify it. Pp. 103–122 in H. Abramson (ed.), *Problems of Consciousness*. New York: Josiah Macy Foundation.

137. READ, G. D. (1933). *Natural Childbirth.* London: Heinemann.

Bibliography

138. READ, G. D. (1955). *Antenatal Illustrated. The Natural Approach to Happy Motherhood*. 2nd edn. 1957. London: Heinemann.

138a. RECHETOVA, L. A. (1961). Rol' jenskikh konsoultatsii v profilaktike riada oslojnienii vo vremia beriemmiennosti i v rodakh (The role of prenatal consultations in the psychoprophylaxis of complications during pregnancy and childbirth). *Voprossi Okhrany Matierinstva i Dietstva*, 4, 82–86 (in Russian).

139. *Revue de Médecine psychosomatique*, special number, 1962. Paris: Maloine.

140. REYNOLDS, P. (1955). Anxiety in pregnancy. *West J. Surg.*, 63, 88–95.

141. ROSENGREN, W. R. (1961). Social sources of pregnancy as illness or abnormality. *Social Forces*, 39, 260–267.

142. ROSENGREN, W. R. (1961). Some social and psychological aspects of delivery room difficulties. *J. nerv. ment. Dis.*, 132, 515–521.

143. SALGANNIK, G. M. (1953). *Rodovaïa Bol i Obezbolivanie (Pains of Childbirth and Analgesia)*. Moscow: Medguiz (in Russian). (French translation of Ch. 2, *Comm. Gynéc. Obstét.*, France-URSS, 1954.)

144. SCOTT, E., and THOMPSON, A. M. (1956). A psychological investigation of primigravidae. IV – Psychological factors and the clinical phenomena of labour. *J. Obstet. Gynaec. Brit. Emp.*, 63, 502–508.

144a. SHLIFER, R. A. (1930). K slovesnomou obezbolivaniou rodovovo akta (Verbal analgesia in childbirth). Pp. 307–318 in *Psikhoterapia*. Kharkov (in Russian).

145. STRAUSS, B. (1956). Mental hygiene in pregnancy. *Amer. J. Nursing*, 56, 314–317.

146. THOMS, H. (1950). *Training for Childbirth: a Program of Natural Childbirth with Rooming-in*. New York: McGraw Hill.

147. *Transcultural psychiatric research review and newsletter* (1963). 14 (April) and 15 (October). Canada.

148. VALABREGA, J. P. (1962). *La relation thérapeutique: malade et médecin*. Paris: Flammarion.

149. VELLAY, P., and CENDRARS, M. (1957). Accouchement sans douleur. *Elle-encyclopédie*. Paris: Fayard.

150. VELLAY, P., and VELLAY, A. (1956). *Témoignages sur l'accouchement sans douleur par la méthode psychoprophylactique*. Paris: Le Seuil.

151. VELVOVSKI, I. Z. (1963). *Sistema Psikhoprofilakticheskovo Obezbolivania Rodov (Psychological Analgesia in Obstetrics)*. Moscow: Gos. Izdat. Med. Lit. (in Russian).

152. VELVOVSKI, I. Z., PLATONOV, K. I., PLOTITCHER, V. A., and CHOUGOM, E. A. (1954). *Psikhoprofilaktika Boliei v Rodakh (Psychoprophylactic Obstetrical Analgesia)* (12 lessons). Leningrad: Medguiz (in Russian). (English version, *Painless Childbirth through Psychoprophylaxis*. Moscow: Foreign Languages Publishing House, 1960.)

153. VERMOREL, H. (1954). *L'accouchement sans douleur par la méthode psychoprophylactique à la lumiere de l'enseignement physiologique de Pavlov*. Lyon: Camugli.

154. VERMOREL, H. (1960). Aspects psychologiques et psychothérapiques dans la méthode psychoprophylactique d'accouchement sans douleur. *Bull. Soc. int. Psychoprophyl. obstét.*, 2, 133–143.

155. WEILL-HALLE, L. (1963). Le rôle du planning familial dans la préparation à la maternité. *Bull. Soc. franç. Psychoprophyl. obstét.*, 15, 57–70.

156. WINOKUR, K. G., and WERBOFF, J. (1956). The relationship of conscious maternal attitudes to certain aspects of pregnancy. *Psychiat. Quart. Suppl.*, 30, 61–73.

157. WORDEN, F. G., and MARSH, J. T. (1963). Amplitude changes of auditory potentials evoked at cochlear nucleus during acoustic habituation. *Electroenceph. clin. Neurophysiol.*, 15, 866–881.

158. ZDRAVOMYSLOV, V. I. (1956). *Obezbolivanie Rodov Vnoucheniem (Obstetrical Analgesia by Suggestion)*. Moscow: Medguiz (in Russian).

Name Index

Figures in parentheses refer to the numbers in the Bibliography

Name Index

296

Subject Index